ADVANCES IN
Cardiac Surgery®

VOLUME 9

ADVANCES IN
Cardiac Surgery®

VOLUME 1 THROUGH 6 (OUT OF PRINT)

ADVANCES IN
Cardiac Surgery®

VOLUME 9

Editor-in-Chief
Robert B. Karp, M.D.
Professor of Surgery, Chief of Cardiac Surgery, University of Chicago,
Pritzker School of Medicine, Chicago, Illinois

Editorial Board
Hillel Laks, M.D.
Professor and Chief, Division of Cardiothoracic Surgery; Director, Heart
Transplant Program, UCLA Medical Center, Los Angeles, California

Andrew S. Wechsler, M.D.
Stuart McGuire Professor and Chairman, Department of Surgery; Chief,
Division of Cardiothoracic Surgery; Professor of Physiology, Medical
College of Virginia, Virginia Commonwealth University, Richmond,
Virginia

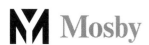 Mosby

St. Louis Baltimore Boston Carlsbad Chicago Naples New York Philadelphia Portland
London Madrid Mexico City Singapore Sydney Tokyo Toronto Wiesbaden

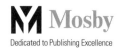

Dedicated to Publishing Excellence

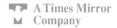
A Times Mirror
Company

Associate Publisher: Cynthia Baudendistel
Developmental Editor: Lulu Danan
Project Manager: Jill C. Waite
Production Project Supervisor: Joy Moore
Production Assistant: Laura Bayless

Printed in the United States of America
Composition by The Clarinda Company
Printing/binding by The Maple-Vail Book Manufacturing Group

Editorial Office:
Mosby–Year Book, Inc.
11830 Westline Industrial Drive
St. Louis, Missouri 63146

International Standard Serial Number: 0889–5074
International Standard Book Number: 0–8151–1849–X

Contributors

Christophe Acar, M.D.
Professor of Cardiac Surgery, Department of Cardiovascular Surgery,
Hôpital Bichat, Paris, France

Juan C. Alejos, M.D.
Assistant Professor of Pediatrics, Division of Cardiology, UCLA Medical
Center, Los Angeles, California

Craig R. Asher, M.D.
Department of Cardiology, The Cleveland Clinic, Cleveland, Ohio

Carl L. Backer, M.D.
Attending Surgeon, Division of Cardiovascular-Thoracic Surgery,
Children's Memorial Hospital; Associate Professor of Surgery,
Northwestern University Medical School, Chicago, Illinois

Federico J. Benetti, M.D.
Fundaciòn Benetti, Buenos Aires, Argentina

Joginder Bhayana, M.D.
Associate Professor of Surgery, Division of Cardiothoracic Surgery,
Buffalo General Hospital and State University of New York at Buffalo,
Buffalo, New York

Mina K. Chung, M.D.
Department of Cardiology, The Cleveland Clinic, Cleveland, Ohio

Kenneth A. Ellenbogen, M.D.
Associate Professor of Medicine, Department of Medicine, Division of
Cardiology, Medical College of Virginia and McGuire VA Medical Center,
Richmond, Virginia

O.H. Frazier, M.D.
Co-Director, Cullen Cardiovascular Research Laboratories; Texas Heart
Institute; Chief, Cardiopulmonary Transplantation, Texas Heart Institute
and St. Luke's Episcopal Hospital; Professor, Department of Surgery,
University of Texas Medical School—Houston, Houston, Texas

Yasuharu Imai, M.D.
Professor and Chairman, Department of Pediatric Cardiovascular
Surgery, The Heart Institute of Japan, Tokyo Women's Medical College,
Tokyo, Japan

Yoichi Kameda, M.D.
Research Associate of Surgery, Department of Surgery III, Nara Medical
College, Kashihara Nara, Japan

Yasunaru Kawashima, M.D.
President Emenitus, National Cardiovascular Center, Suita, Osaka, Japan

James K. Kirklin, M.D.
Professor, Department of Surgery, Division of Cardiothoracic Surgery,
University of Alabama, Birmingham, Alabama

Soichiro Kitamura, M.D.
Professor of Surgery, Department of Surgery III, Nara Medical College,
Kashihara Nara, Japan

Hillel Laks, M.D.
Professor and Chief, Division of Cardiothoracic Surgery, Director, Heart
Transplant Program, UCLA Medical Center, Los Angeles, California

Gianfranco Lisi, M.D.
Istituto di Chirurgia Toracica e Cardiovascolare, Università di Siena,
Siena, Italy

Massimo Maccherini, M.D.
Istituto di Chirurgia Toracica e Cardiovascolare, Università di Siena,
Siena, Italy

S. Katie Mackey, R.N.
Clinical Studies Coordinator, International Heart Institute of Montana
Foundation, Missoula, Montana

Massimo A. Mariani, M.D.
Istituto di Chirurgia Toracica e Cardiovascolare, Università di Siena,
Siena, Italy

Constantine Mavroudis, M.D.
Head, Division of Cardiovascular-Thoracic Surgery, Children's Memorial
Hospital; Professor of Surgery, Northwestern University Medical School,
Chicago, Illinois

David C. McGiffin, M.D.
Associate Professor, Department of Surgery, Division of Cardiothoracic
Surgery, University of Alabama, Birmingham, Alabama

Noel L. Mills, M.D.
Professor of Surgery, Tulane University School of Medicine, New Orleans, Louisiana

Patrick Nataf, M.D.
Service de Chirurgie Cardiaque, Hôpital de la Pitié, Paris, France

James H. Oury, M.D.
Director of Cardiovascular Services, International Heart Institute of Montana Foundation, Missoula, Montana

F. Bennett Pearce, M.D.
Assistant Professor, Department of Pediatrics, Division of Cardiology, University of Alabama, Birmingham, Alabama

Tomas A. Salerno, M.D.
Professor of Surgery, Chief of Cardiothoracic Surgery, Division of Cardiothoracic Surgery, Buffalo General Hospital and State University of New York at Buffalo, Buffalo, New York

Guido Sani, M.D.
Professore di Chirurgia Cardìaco, Istituto di Chirurgia Toracica e Cardiovascolare, Università di Siena, Siena, Italy

Frank G. Scholl, M.D.
Research Fellow, Division of Cardiothoracic Surgery, UCLA Medical Center, Los Angeles, California

Michele Toscano, M.D.
Istituto di Chirurgia Toracica e Cardiovascolare, Università di Siena, Siena, Italy

Mark A. Wood, M.D.
Assistant Professor of Medicine, Department of Medicine, Division of Cardiology, Medical College of Virginia and McGuire VA Medical Center, Richmond, Virginia

Contents

Arterial Grafts for Coronary Artery Bypass.

CHAPTER 1

Mitral Valve Homograft

Christophe Acar, M.D.
Professor of Cardiac Surgery, Department of Cardiovascular Surgery,
Hopital Bichat, Paris, France

HISTORICAL BACKGROUND

T he first animal experiments with orthotopic heart valve transplantation involved the tricuspid valve and were performed by Robicsek in 1951.[1]

In the early 1960s, transplantation of the mitral valve was the subject of a number of animal studies (Bernhard et al.,[2] Cachera et al.,[3] Hubka et al.,[4] O'Brien and Gerbode,[5] Rastelli et al.,[6] and Van Vliet et al.[7]). Early valve failure was demonstrated in most cases. However, some animals survived with a good valvular function and were followed for a period of up to 3 years.[5, 7] Histologic studies in survivors assessed the healing process of the mitral homograft with time.[8] It has been interesting to observe the rapidity with which the papillary muscle remained strongly attached to the ventricular myocardium.[9]

Histologic studies in transplanted valves showed that the muscular portion of the graft promptly underwent ischemic necrosis and replacement by fibrotic tissue derived from adjacent host tissue.[4, 8, 9] Dense scar tissue was present 6 months after implantation, and sporadic areas of viable myocardium most likely corresponded to remnants of the native papillary muscle.

In 1965, Senning performed the first mitral homograft in a patient.[10] Mitral homografts were used to replace either the mitral or the tricuspid valve in 11 cases. The papillary muscles were buried into a trench created in the recipient muscles. Early valve failure occurred, and all patients underwent reoperation within 3 years. During the same time, Ross[11] and Yacoub and Kittle[12] attempted to replace the mitral valve using a semilunar homograft, with disappointing midterm results.

More recently, at the University of Kiel, Bernhard used an antibiotic-preserved mitral homograft in three cases for mitral valve replacement. The technique of papillary muscle insertion was modified using a transmural suture through the ventricular wall (transpapillary muscle extracardiac epicardial fixation[13]). Early chordal rupture occurred within the first postoperative year caused by technical error or by endocarditis.[14] One patient had a stable result for 4 years until rupture of the scarred papillary muscle occurred requiring reoperation.[14]

A few years ago, Pomar and Mestres reported their experience with the use of mitral homografts for tricuspid valve endocarditis in three patients who were drug addicts.[15] Encouraged by their experience, we decided to apply general principles established by Carpentier for mitral valve reconstruction[16] to the use of homografts for mitral valve replacement.

A preliminary experimental study was performed in eight goats. The papillary muscles of the graft were selectively treated by immersion into glutaraldehyde for 40 minutes to facilitate their insertion. After 6 months, calcifications involving the chordae at their attachment on the papillary muscle were noted. Consequently, glutaraldehyde fixation of the papillary muscles was subsequently abandoned in the clinical series.

In 1992, a cryopreserved mitral homograft was successfully inserted in a patient with calcified rheumatic stenosis.[17] Since then, we have reevaluated the use of either partial or total mitral homograft replacement in 61 patients.[18-20]

HOMOGRAFT PROCUREMENT

In France, the availability of homografts harvested in postmortem donors is poor because of legal restrictions. All mitral homografts were obtained from beating hearts; the valves were harvested either in brain dead patients considered to be unsuitable heart donors or in recipient's hearts explanted at the time of tranplantation.[20] The mitral valve of transplant recipients was collected as a homograft provided that it was anatomically normal. Ischemic heart disease was not considered as a contraindication for valve storage, even in case of a fibrotic papillary muscle.

The entire mitral valve apparatus was dissected free including both the attachment of the papillary muscles onto the ventricular wall and the myocardium surrounding the mitral annulus. Care was taken in dissection of the aorto-mitral triangular area to ensure that an aortic homograft could also be harvested. This dissection was performed in a sterile theater. Cryopreservation was performed within 18 hours of retrieval of the homograft in the Tissue Bank of Hospital St. Louis, in Paris.

A preservative solution containing 5% dimethyl sulfoxide without antibiotics was used, and the temperature was gradually decreased using vaporized nitrogen to $-150°$ C. The homograft was stored in nitrogen until its use.

CLASSIFICATION OF THE PAPILLARY MUSCLES

At first glance, papillary muscles appear as random formations escaping any categorization. However, close observations have revealed the existence of anatomical patterns as well as insertional modalities that reappear regularly.

Careful examination of the anatomy of the papillary muscles in 68 hearts confirmed our clinical perception of the existence of a correspondence between the papillary muscle division and the chordae's mode of attachment to the leaflets. We thus established a classification irrespective of the shape that takes only into account the existence of a dividing plane and the relationship between the papillary muscle and the leaflets.[20] Four types of increasing complexity were distinguished (Fig 1):

Type I. The papillary muscle is undivided. It gives rise to all chordae tendineae, which fan out to the corresponding hemivalves. Type I is the most common presentation and accounts for 63% of the anterolateral and 41% of the posteromedial muscle (Fig 1, A).

Type II. The papillary muscle is divided in a sagittal plane into two heads. One head supports exclusively the posterior leaflet. The other is related to the commissural region and to the anterior leaflet. This type is observed in 7% of the anterolateral and in 39% of the posteromedial papillary muscle (Fig 1, B).

Type III. The papillary muscle is divided in a coronal plane into two or more heads. A single head relates exclusively to the commissural zone. The remaining heads support the chordae to the anterior and to the posterior leaflets. The different heads originate from the same level on the ventricular wall. The proportions are 15% for the anterolateral and 7% for the posteromedial papillary muscle (Fig 1, C).

Type IV. The papillary muscle is complex and is characterized by division in a coronal plane and by staged origin of the different heads. One tiny muscular band close to the annulus gives insertion to commissural chordae. As a result, the latter are invariably short. The rest of the papillary muscle, which may be single or divided, is located at a lower level on the ventricular wall and supports the rest of the leaflet. This type represents 15% of the anterolateral and 13% of the posteromedial papillary muscle (Fig 1, D).

In all hearts examined, we could easily identify the four types

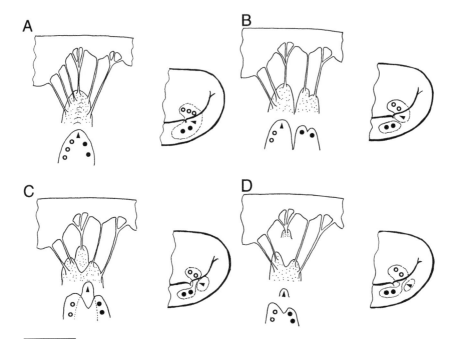

FIGURE 1.
Morphologic classification of papillary muscles. Note that the commissural chord invariably arises from the tip of the papillary muscle. **A,** Type I: simple, single muscle. **B,** type II: division in the sagittal plane forming an individual head supporting the posterior leaflet. **C,** type III: division in the coronal plane forming an individual head supporting a commissure. **D,** type IV: divisions with multiple levels of origin from the ventricular wall. Short commissural chordae inserted on an isolated muscular band, and the remaining head originates at a lower level on the ventricle. ▲, commissural chord; ○, chord to anterior leaflet; •, chord to posterior leaflet.

without difficulty. Intermediate cases exist, in which one may hesitate deciding between types II and III or between III and IV. However, by following the guidelines described, one can always classify an apparently ambiguous form.

Type I is easy to handle as well as type II and III as long as the orientation of the separate heads are preserved. Type IV, however, raises important technical difficulties and should be discarded. The morphologic type of each papillary muscle should be indicated on the homograft identification card to enable the surgeon to be more specific about his choice.

VALVE SIZING AND GRAFT SELECTION

Whereas the cylindrical form of the aortic valve allows its size to be measured by the transverse diameter of the orifice as the sole measurement, the evaluation of the dimensions of the mitral valve is more difficult. Both the extent of valvular leaflet tissue and that of the subvalvular apparatus must be taken into consideration.

In our series, the measurement chosen to size the leaflet tissue of the valve was the height of the anterior leaflet tissue in its mid-portion. This measurement was obtained in the recipient by trans-esophageal echocardiography using a sagittal section of the mitral orifice passing through the papillary muscles and aortic orifice (Fig 2, A). The height of the leaflet was measured in the open position (diastole) so as to clearly identify the free edge of the valve. The same parameter was obtained for the homograft by direct measurement of the valve (Fig 2, B).

A good estimate of the size of the subvalvular apparatus could be obtained by measuring the distance between the annulus and the apex of the papillary muscle. This parameter is not directly affected by any pathologic process involving the valve. It has the advantage of taking into consideration ventricular dilatation if present, which would indicate the need for a larger homograft. This parameter can be obtained using both direct measurement of the homograft and echocardiographic study of the patient's valve.

The identification card of the mitral homograft included the different measurements (height of the anterior leaflet, distance between papillary muscles and annulus). To obtain an optimal sizing, echocardiographic measurements of the valve were matched with those of the identification card of the homograft. A homograft 3-mm larger than the valve was selected to provide slight excess tissue and offer a large surface of coaptation.

SURGICAL TECHNIQUE

PREPARATION OF THE GRAFT

The homograft was prepared before cardiopulmonary bypass was instituted. The homograft was thawed in the operating room at 40° C and then rinsed in 5% dextrose solution. First, the atrial muscle inserted to the annulus of the valve was dissected off. Then the wall of the left ventricle attached to the annulus was excised without traumatizing the valve tissue, particularly in the commissural areas. The connective tissue of the right and left trigones, which were frequently the site of a fibrocalcareous nodule, was trimmed. Finally, the fatty tissue in the atrioventricular junction was removed.

Before preparing the papillary muscles, their morphology was examined and noted to ensure that the orientation would be maintained at the time of implantation. Each papillary muscle was detached from its insertion into the ventricular wall, leaving approxi-

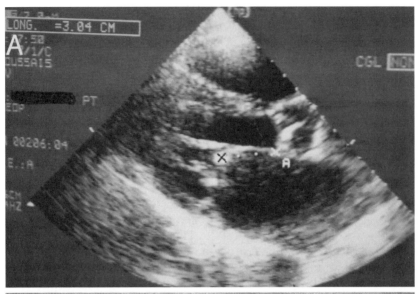

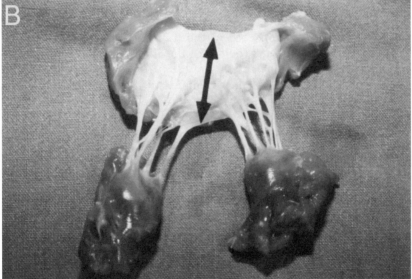

FIGURE 2.
Valve sizing. **A,** echocardiographic measurement of the anterior leaflet in diastole using a sagittal view; aortic valve and papillary muscles were visible. **B,** Direct measurement of the height of the homograft anterior leaflet. A homograft slightly larger than the valve is selected.

mately 15 mm of muscular tissue beyond the origin of the chordae. The valve was then placed in a container of 5% dextrose until its use.

Myocardial protection was achieved using cold cardioplegia injected into the aortic root. The left atrium was approached via the classic parallel incision in the interatrial sulcus. The mitral valve was inspected to assess the pathologic process and to decide which operative technique would be necessary. In the presence of an isolated lesion affecting less than half of the valve (calcification or valvular abscess), a partial homograft was inserted provided that the remainder of the valve was normal. On the other hand, in the presence of extensive lesions involving the entire valve, total homograft replacement was performed.

FIXATION OF THE PAPILLARY MUSCLES

First, the pathologic valve tissue was excised and the relevant chordae divided at their insertion. Contrary to various methods described in the literature[10, 13, 15] that use an end-to-end fixation of homograft to native papillary muscles, we have adopted a different approach using a side-to-side suture of the papillary muscles.[18]

The papillary muscle of the recipient was not amputated, so that the maximum amount of viable myocardium remained to support the homograft. These were mobilized by dividing the muscular bands attaching them to the ventricular wall. The homograft implantation was then commenced by fixation of the papillary muscles, starting with the posterior one. The exposure of the recipient papillary muscle was optimized by applying gentle traction on a stay-suture placed at this level. Each homograft papillary muscle was inserted into the slit between the native papillary muscle and the wall of the left ventricle (Fig 3). Great care was taken to maintain the respective positions of the different heads to obtain an even distribution of traction on the leaflet tissue. The head supporting the commissure was used as a reference point and was positioned at the corresponding site on the native papillary muscle. This site was easily identified because the commissural chordae invariably originate from the apex of the papillary muscle.

As a general rule, the papillary muscle of the homograft was sutured side-to-side at a slightly lower level on the recipient. A double row of sutures was used to implant the papillary muscle. First, several mattress sutures were placed at the base of the graft papillary muscle. Second, multiple interrupted sutures were placed around the margins of the graft. Finally, the apex was used to attach it firmly to the native papillary muscle. The sutures were placed so as not to interfere with the origin of the chordae because this could eventually lead to chordal erosion. At the level of emergence of the cords, the problem was avoided by using mattress sutures.

No material was used to reinforce the suture whether prosthetic (Teflon or polytetryfluoroethylene)[13, 21, 22, 23] or biological (pericardium).[23] Based on experience acquired through the technique of chordal shortening described by Carpentier,[16] it is our belief that the use of foreign material at the point of origin of the cords can weaken their insertion and induce an appreciable risk of chordal erosion.

The reliability of the technique of implantation used in this study depends on the healing process of the papillary muscles with progressive replacement with fibrotic tissue. This method contrasts with a purely mechanical approach using interposition of prosthetic material and/or transfixing stitches through the ventricular wall to counteract the physical stress.

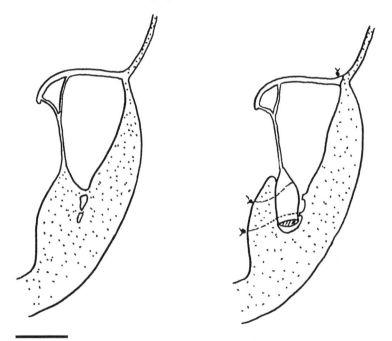

FIGURE 3.
Papillary muscle implantation. The trabeculae attaching the papillary muscle to the ventricle are divided. The graft's papillary muscle is sutured side-to-side into the trench created between the papillary muscle and the ventricle.

FIXATION OF THE LEAFLET TISSUE AND RING ANNULOPLASTY

The homograft leaflet tissue was then sutured circumferentially to the mitral annulus using continuous 5/0 prolene. The various portions of the valve were attached in the following order: (1) posteromedial commissure, (2) anterior leaflet, (3) anterolateral commissure, and (4) posterior leaflet. Particular attention was taken in positioning the commissures, and the suture was effected without tension in the areas of the anterior leaflet and commissures. In cases of excess or deficient homograft leaflet tissue with respect to the mitral annulus, the suturing style was modified to achieve equilibration while attaching the posterior leaflet.

Ring annuloplasty was systematically performed in all cases of mitral homograft.[20] The sutures for the annuloplasty ring were placed before the valve leaflet tissue was attached. The size of annuloplasty ring was chosen according to the size of the anterior leaflet of the homograft, measured with an obturator. The use of an annuloplasty ring provides many advantages: (1) it permits, precise adaptation of the size of the annulus to that of the homograft; (2) the ring absorbs some of the mechanical stress exerted by ventricular contraction and alleviates traction that would otherwise be directly applied on the valvular suture line; and (3) ring annuloplasty allows a greater surface of leaflet coaptation, thereby lowering the tension on the subvalvular apparatus. The slight overcorrection achieved by annuloplasty may compensate for imperfections in the regulation of tension of the chordae. The final result was evaluated by infusion of saline under pressure into the ventricle.

PARTIAL MITRAL HOMOGRAFT

The idea to partially replace the mitral valve with a portion of homograft is not new (Fig 4). In 1964, Cachera et al. introduced the concept of partial homograft replacement.[3] He studied varied techniques of mitral valvuloplasty: (1) grafting of a patch of homologous leaflet tissue; (2) replacement of the entire anterior leaflet with its subvalvular apparatus using the corresponding portion of a homograft; and (3) total homograft replacement.[3] More recently, Revuelta et al., in a study using an animal model and scanning electron microscopy, demonstrated the perfect integration of a partial homograft when placed amid native mitral tissue.[9]

Use of a partial mitral homograft should be considered as part of the wide range of techniques of mitral valve repair. It is technically feasible to reconstitute a portion of mitral valve leaflet tissue

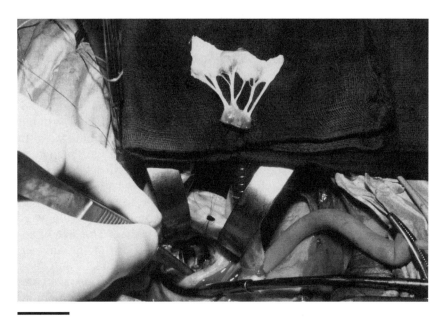

FIGURE 4.
Partial mitral homograft.

using biological material (autologous pericardium), and it is also possible to replace several chordae either using chordal transposition or prosthetic chordae.[16, 24] However, the presence of a voluminous pathologic process that affects both leaflet tissue and chordae, especially when involving a commissural region, represents a serious limitation to valve reconstruction. This situation is met most frequently in two conditions: mitral stenosis with calcification and acute bacterial endocarditis with localized abscess formation and vegetations. The remainder of the valve must be normal because a pathologic remnant may lead to a mediocre result.[20]

Technically, it seems preferable to divide the valve vertically with the aim of replacing a commissural region or a hemivalve, rather than dividing the valve along the horizontal axis and achieving replacement of an entire leaflet. A vertical division allows selective replacement of 25% to 50% of the valve according to the extent of the lesions. A distinct advantage is that only one papillary muscle needs to be reimplanted. Also, valvular closure results from coaptation between two leaflets of the same origin belonging either to the homograft or to the native valve.

Transplantation of an entire leaflet does not appear to be a fully satisfactory procedure and presents certain drawbacks. Both papillary muscles must be reimplanted and exposure is made more difficult by the presence of the opposing leaflet and its cords. Afterwards, the presence of a suture line in the region of the commissures can potentially impair the opening of the valve. Furthermore, valve closure results from apposition between the homograft and the opposite native leaflet, and the mildest asymmetry in chordal tension may lead to relative prolapse. We no longer recommend its use, and in the presence of lesions invading a whole leaflet, total replacement of the mitral valve is accomplished.

PATIENT POPULATION

INDICATIONS

Since 1992, 61 patients aged 10–73 years (mean age, 41 $\pm$ 5 years) underwent partial ($n = 24$) or total ($n = 37$) mitral valve replacement with a cryopreserved homograft. The indications for operation were rheumatic mitral stenosis ($n = 37$), acute infective endocarditis ($n = 20$), degenerative mitral insufficiency ($n = 2$), and systemic lupus ($n = 2$). Most patients were in sinus rhythm, and 14 patients undergoing total homograft insertion were having repeat operations.

RESULTS

There were three early deaths resulting from severe biventricular failure despite normally functioning homografts. These patients had severe preoperative contractile dysfunction and had undergone multiple reoperations.

One elderly patient required an early reoperation at 10 days. This patient had a staphylococcal bacterial endocarditis on a Starr Edwards mitral prosthesis that we attempted to replace with a homograft. Initial echocardiography was satisfactory, but a rapid deterioration occured at 10 days requiring reoperation. There was a dehiscence of the homograft at the suture line attaching the leaflet tissue to the annulus in the region of the anterior commissure, probably caused by excess traction on the cords. After reoperation, the patient had an uneventful recovery. In general, the insertion of a mitral homograft for replacement of a prosthetic valve has not been satisfactory (one death and one early reoperation). All other patients had uneventful postoperative courses.

All patients were reviewed after a follow-up of up to 4 years. One patient died at 5 months from lung carcinoma. Two patients with partial homograft replacement required reoperation at 16 and 18 months, respectively. The causes of reoperation were residual stenosis resulting from fibrosis of the native valve in one case and recurrence of endocarditis in the other case. All 53 remaining patients had normal functional status, (New York Heart Association I or II), and most of them were in sinus rhythm with no medical treatment.

Echocardiography at a mean follow-up of 23 months revealed stable results when compared with intraoperative echocardiography. There was no case with moderate or severe insufficiency. The transvalvular gradient was 3 ± 4 mm Hg, and the surface valve area measured by planimetry was 2.5 ± 3 cm^2.

REFERENCES

1. Robicsek F, Sanger PW, Taylor FH, et al: Transplantability of heart valves. *Arch Surg* 84:141–148, 1962.
2. Bernhard VA, Ringdal R, Babotai I, et al: Zur Homotransplantation der Mitralklappe technik und postoperative funktionelle Resultate. *Thoraxchirurgie* 13:89–95, 1965.
3. Cachera JP, Salvatore L, Hermant J, et al: Reconstructions plastiques de l'appareil mitral chez le chien au moyen de valves mitrales homologues conservées. *Ann Chir Thorac Cardiovasc* 3:459–474, 1964.
4. Hubka M, Siska K, Brozman M, et al: Replacement of mitral and tricuspid valves by mitral homograft. *J Thorac Cardiovasc Surg* 51:195–204, 1966.
5. O'Brien MF, Gerbode F: Homotransplantation of the mitral valve: Preliminary experimental report and review of the literature. *Aust N Z J Surg* 34:81–88, 1964.
6. Rastelli GC, Berghuis J, Swan HJC: Evaluation of function of mitral valve after homotransplantation in the dog. *J Thorac Cardiovasc Surg* 49:459–474, 1965.
7. Van Vliet PD, Titus JL, Berghuis J, et al: Morphologic features of homotransplanted canine mitral valves. *J Thorac Cardiovasc Surg* 49:504–510, 1965.
8. Tamura K, Jones M, Yamada I, et al: A comparison of failure modes of glutaraldehyde-treated versus antibiotic-prserved mitral valve allografts implanted in sheep. *J Thorac Cardiovasc Surg* 110:224–238, 1994.
9. Revuelta JM, Cagigas JC, Bernal JM, et al: Partial replacement of the mitral valve by homografts: An experimental study. *J Thorac Cardiovasc Surg* 104:1274–1279, 1992.
10. Senning A: Rekonstruktion der Mitralklappe: Homoioplastik. *Thoraxchir Vask Chir* 16:601–605, 1968.
11. Ross DN: Replacement of the aortic and mitral valves with a pulmonary autograft. *Lancet* 2:956, 1967.
12. Yacoub MH, Kittle C: A new technique for replacement of the mitral valve by a semilunar valve homograft. *J Thorac Cardiovasc Surg* 58:859–869, 1969.

13. Sievers HH, Lange PE, Yankah AC, et al: Allogeneous transplantation of the mitral valve: An open question. *Thorac Cardiovasc Surg* 33:227–229, 1986.
14. Yankah AC, Sievers HH, Lange PE, et al: Clinical report on stentless mitral allografts. *J Heart Valve Dis* 4:40–44, 1995.
15. Pomar JL, Mestres CA: Tricuspid valve replacement using a mitral homograft: surgical technique and initial results. *J Heart Valve Dis* 2:125–128, 1993.
16. Carpentier A: Mitral valve repair: The French "correction." *J Thorac Cardiovasc Surg* 86:323–337, 1983.
17. Acar C, Farge A, Ramsheyi A, et al: Mitral valve replacement using a cryopreserved mitral homograft. *Ann Thorac Surg* 57:746–748, 1994.
18. Acar C, Gaer J, Chauvaud S, et al: Technique of homograft replacement of the mitral valve. *J Heart Valve Dis* 4:31–34, 1995.
19. Acar C, Iung B, Cormier B, et al: Double mitral homograft for recurrent bacterial endocarditis of the tricuspid and mitral valves. *J Heart Valve Dis* 3:470–472, 1994.
20. Acar C, Tolan M, Berrebi A, et al: Homograft replacement of the mitral valve: Graft selection, technique of implantation and results in forty-three patients. *J Thorac Cardiovasc Surg* 111:367–380, 1996.
21. Kumar AS, Chander H, Trehan H: Surgical technique of multiple valve replacement with biological valves: A new option. *J Heart Valve Dis* 4:45–46, 1995.
22. Kumar AS, Trehan H: Homograft mitral valve replacement: A case report. *J Heart Valve Dis* 3:473–475, 1994.
23. Vetter HO, Dagge A, Liao K, et al: Mitral allograft with chordal support: Echocardiographic evaluation in sheep. *J Heart Valve Dis* 4:35–39, 1995.
24. Frater RWM, Vetter HO, Zussa C, et al: Chordal replacement in mitral valve repair. *Circulation* 82:125–130, 1992.

CHAPTER 2

Pulmonary Autografts

James H. Oury, M.D.
Director of Cardiovascular Services, International Heart Institute of Montana Foundation, Missoula, Montana

S. Katie Mackey, R.N.
Clinical Studies Coordinator, International Heart Institute of Montana Foundation, Missoula, Montana

T he search for the perfect aortic valve replacement continues because limitations still plague both mechanical and bioprosthetic valves.[1-3] Replacement of the aortic root with the pulmonary autograft in patients with isolated aortic root pathology provides an excellent alternative to replacement with a mechanical, bioprosthetic, or allograft valve. Hemodynamic function is optimized because the pulmonary autograft offers characteristics inherent in the native aortic valve. These characteristics, as well as the pulmonary autograft's proven long-term integrity as a living tissue valve, have made it an attractive alternative for young individuals with aortic valve disease.

It was the experimental work of Lower et al.[4, 5] in 1961 and Pillsbury and Shumway[6] in 1966 that demonstrated the feasibility of transferring the pulmonary valve into the aortic position. This work led Ross to pursue the concept of the pulmonary autograft procedure, with the first successful clinical application of the pulmonary autograft in the aortic position occurring under his direction in 1967.[7] In 1988, Ross published his personal series encompassing his results with the procedure from 1967 to 1986.[8] These encouraging results based primarily on improved myocardial protection, a heightened awareness of coronary anatomy, and experimental evidence confirming the durability of the pulmonary valve in the aortic position prompted renewed interest in this procedure. In spite of these promising indications, the pulmonary autograft procedure was slow to meet universal acceptance because of its inherent complexity and the necessity of a two-valve procedure to treat single-valve pathology.

INTERNATIONAL REGISTRY OF THE ROSS (PULMONARY AUTOGRAFT) PROCEDURE

The Ross Registry was established in 1993 after the First Annual Ross Colloquium, held at the time of the American Association for Thoracic Surgery (AATS) meeting in Chicago. Although Ross' results suggested that the pulmonary autograft procedure might be a lifelong solution to aortic valve disease that requires valve replacement, it seemed appropriate to make a concerted effort to establish a multicenter, long-term follow-up study to examine longitudinal clinical outcomes associated with the procedure, as well as attempt to resolve and identify the many technical considerations necessary for successful execution of the procedure. It was with these issues in mind that the Ross Registry was established. The purpose of the registry is threefold:

1. to identify through the registry all cardiac surgeons in the world who currently perform the procedure;
2. to investigate and track the technical details associated with the procedure as they develop;
3. and to register all Ross procedures performed worldwide, both retrospectively and prospectively, and follow these long-term patient outcomes over time.

The Ross Registry was simple in design and included completion of two 1-page case report forms. The initial form tracks patient demographics, medical history, and technical considerations of the procedure and is completed at the time of surgery. The follow-up form is completed 6 months postoperatively, and annually thereafter, to capture long-term patient outcomes in terms of freedom from reoperation, freedom from autograft failure, and freedom from death. Aggregate data from the Ross Registry are compiled annually in an International Summary Report that is shared with all surgeons participating in the Registry. In addition, participating surgeons receive individual reports outlining the data from their personal series. This allows comparison with the International Summary Report and identification of trends within each physician-patient series.

At present, the International Registry of the Ross Procedure identifies 126 surgeons worldwide who perform the procedure. The exponential growth of the procedure is illustrated in Figure 1.

PULMONARY AUTOGRAFT PROCEDURE

ADVANTAGES

The pulmonary autograft procedure offers some distinct advantages over other valve replacement alternatives. The primary

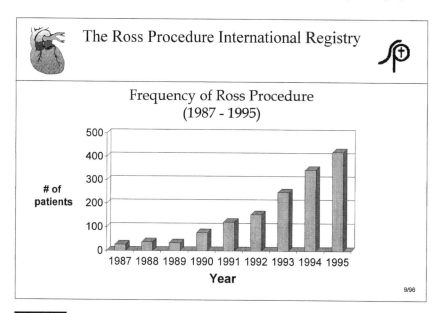

The Ross Procedure International Registry

Frequency of Ross Procedure
(1987 - 1995)

9/96

FIGURE 1.

Exponential growth of the Ross procedure from 1987 to 1995.

advantage inherent in the procedure is that the pulmonary autograft mimics the intrinsic structural characteristics of the native aortic valve.[9] Because the pulmonary autograft is living tissue native to the patient, the threat of thrombus formation is greatly reduced, as is the need for long-term anticoagulation therapy. Its hemodynamic superiority as compared with other replacement devices, be it mechanical or bioprosthetic, is also partly the result of its similarity to the normal human aortic valve. Long-term viability of pulmonary valve autografts have been demonstrated, and they appear more resistant to deterioration than aortic allografts.[10]

In examining the outcome of the right ventricular outflow tract (RVOT) reconstruction, the failure rate (revision or replacement of the pulmonary homograft) reported from 1987 to the present as documented in the Ross Registry is 1.1%. This compares favorably with Ross' personal series in which the RVOT revision rate is 12% during 20 years of follow-up.[8] Several technical developments may have contributed to the decrease in RVOT failure. Improved standardization, modern harvesting methods, and advanced preservation techniques have resulted in the increased availability of an improved homograft. Although initial results in the Ross Registry ap-

TABLE 1.

Current Indications for Aortic Valve Replacement
With a Pulmonary Autograft

- Patient between 11 and 50 years of age (male or female)
- Isolated aortic valve pathology (male or female)
- Endocarditis limited to the aortic root
- Athlete or young individual in whom anticoaulation is contraindicated and optimal hemodynamics are desirable

pear promising in terms of the fate of RVOT reconstruction, more long-term follow-up is necessary to confirm these results.

The pulmonary autograft has demonstrated the potential for growth. This represents a distinct advantage for children and young adults in terms of aortic valve replacement options.[11]

The long-term valve survival of the pulmonary autograft exceeds that of other valve replacement alternatives, which include homografts, porcine, and mechanical valves.[12] Ross et al.[13] have reviewed their long-term results after the procedure in 339 patients followed up for as many as 24 years and found that, 20 years after the procedure, 80% of patients were alive, 85% of this population had not required reoperation, and 75% were free from any other event, including endocarditis, degeneration of the pulmonary autograft, reoperation, and death.

The obvious advantages of the pulmonary autograft procedure when compared with the alternatives for aortic valve replacement must be tempered by the fact that the procedure is technically complex and is accompanied by a steep learning curve even in the most experienced surgeons' hands. This technical complexity is manifest by the fact that the procedure involves a two-valve surgical procedure to repair single aortic valve pathology.

INDICATIONS

The indications for the pulmonary autograft procedure have broadened over time primarily because of the increased availability of commercially cyropreserved aortic valves and their pulmonary valve allograft counterpart, as well as the development of safe techniques for the replacement of the aortic root[8, 10, 14] and increasing familiarity with the procedure. Current indications for the procedure are outlined in Table 1.

First and foremost, the pulmonary autograft procedure is designed for the young patient who has aortic valve disease. The accepted age range for patients having the pulmonary autograft procedure has expanded significantly. The mean age for patients enrolled in the Registry is 29 years (range, 1 day to 73 years). The probable reasons for this expanding age consideration are twofold. First, early mortality for the operation has decreased as evidenced by the results in the Registry. A comparison of the mortality data from Ross' original series and all cases reported in the Registry from 1987 to the present indicate that both early and late mortality have decreased, from 6.6% to 2.3% and from 7.45% to 2.0%, respectively.[8] Second, relative to the growth potential of the pulmonary autograft and success of the operation in children,[11, 15] many surgeons view the procedure as a solution for congenital aortic stenosis that can be performed early in life, and possibly eliminate the need for multiple aortic valve replacements. As increasing durability of the operation is evidenced, older patients with more active lifestyles become candidates for the procedure.

Although sex is not a significant variable in terms of patient outcome or selection, the pulmonary autograft procedure is certainly indicated for young women of childbearing potential. This relates primarily to the problems associated with the use of warfarin during pregnancy. Studies have shown that the use of warfarin during the first trimester of pregnancy can cause craniofacial abnormalities, congenital heart disease, and retardation. Exposure to the drug in both the second and third trimester of pregnancy also results in birth defects and may cause prematurity and stillbirth.[16]

One area where the pulmonary autograft procedure is gaining wider acceptance and application is in patients who have acute bacterial endocarditis. Although it is too early to venture whether the pulmonary autograft will be more resistant to infection than prosthetic valves in the long term, early data suggest that the reinfection rate for autografts is lower than that reported for bioprosthetic valves, mechanical valves, and aortic homografts.[17] Individual series presented by Joyce et al.[18] and Oswalt and Dewan[19] also confirm these encouraging early outcomes.

Special consideration should be given to athletes who need aortic valve replacement. Because of the kinds of activities in which they participate, athletes are often not in a position to subject themselves to the risks inherent in anticoagulation that accompanies most valve replacement alternatives. In addition, these individuals often experience extreme levels of physical activity in pursuit of their athletic activities. These two factors make the pulmonary autograft the optimal choice for aortic valve replacement in this cohort. Exercise stress testing was used to obtain preliminary exercise data from 14 conditioned athletes[20] who had all undergone the Ross procedure. These data were compared with data from 14 normal athletes of similar age using the same exercise testing protocol, which evaluated these athletes across a broad range of exercise conditions (resting to maximum exertion). Results indicate that the Ross athletes exhibited normal hemodynamics as evidenced by physiologic aortic valve gradients and normal echocardiographic profiles to peak exercise levels when compared with the normal control athletes.

The indications for the Ross procedure continue to expand as familiarity with the procedure increases and as long-term outcomes continue to be favorable. When considering a patient for the procedure, the two issues that must be kept in mind are the attendant risks associated with anticoagulation and the hemodynamic consequences of prosthetic devices. In lieu of these considerations, appropriate patient selection continues to be the active patient whose life expectancy exceeds 20 years, and the patient whose lifestyle choices make the pulmonary autograft the optimal alternative.

CONTRAINDICATIONS

As indications for the pulmonary autograft expand, contraindications decrease. However, absolute and relative contraindications continue to exist and are listed in Table 2. Although in some cases these contraindications are subjective, they are widely and generally accepted.

In general, the patient who has multivessel coronary artery disease would not be an appropriate candidate for the pulmonary autograft procedure. Relative to the inherent complexity involved with this operation, and the often prolonged ischemic time, a more

TABLE 2.
Current Absolute Contraindications for Aortic Valve Replacement With the Pulmonary Autograft

- Advanced-vessel coronary artery disease
- Extreme age (younger than 1 year or older than 70 years)
- Extensive multivalve pathology necessitating replacement
- Severely decreased left ventricular function
- Marfan syndrome
- Multisystem organ failure (pulmonary, renal, hepatic, etc.)
- Pulmonary valve pathology (congenital, acquired, iatrogenic)

expeditious implantation should be used in the setting of severe coronary artery disease.

It would appear that the pulmonary autograft procedure would be contraindicated in both the extremely young and those of advanced age. Although initial results from the Ross Registry indicate successful application of this procedure to both extremes of age and the growth of the pulmonary autograft has been documented experimentally,[21] more follow-up is needed to validate long-term clinical outcomes.

Multivalve pathology is considered a contraindication to the Ross procedure, especially in terms of the prolonged ischemic time a multiple valve replacement operation would require. The exception to this would be the instance where the surgeon can predict with confidence that a mitral or tricuspid valve repair done in concert with the pulmonary autograft procedure would provide the patient with a favorable long-term result.

Patients who have diminished left ventricular function (less than 30%), although not an absolute contraindication, should be judged on an individual basis in terms of appropriateness of application of the procedure. Two variables to examine in terms of decreased left ventricular function when determining patient selection for the procedure are the pathologic events and the time frame leading up to presentation, considered in conjunction with the possibility of reversibility.

Application of the Ross procedure to those patients with rheumatic aortic valve disease has been questioned by Kumar et al.[22] In examining a young rheumatic population that has undergone the Ross procedure, echocardiographic data have demonstrated progressive aortic insufficiency in 37 patients followed for more than 6 months postoperatively. The long-term outcome of active rheumatic disease on the viability of the pulmonary autograft remains to be evaluated.

Patients with Marfan syndrome are not appropriate candidates for the Ross procedure. The pulmonary root is not a satisfactory substitute for the aortic root in these patients because the generalized connective tissue abnormalities intrinsic in this disorder are also present in the pulmonary artery, as well as the aortic cusps. This has been reported in the literature in cases in which autograft replacement of the aortic valve in a patient with Marfan syndrome resulted in progressive and fatal bleeding. Marfan histology was confirmed by histologic examination of the excised pulmonary valve, which demonstrated medial necrosis of the pulmonary artery and myxomatous degeneration of the valve.[23]

Patients who have multisystem organ failure are also not candidates for the pulmonary autograft procedure, primarily because of the often prolonged intraoperative course that the technical complexity of the procedure mandates. The resulting systemic effects of prolonged coronary pulmonary bypass on an already compromised patient reinforce organ failure as a contraindication to the procedure.

The intraoperative discovery of a native pulmonary valve deformity, whether congenital, acquired, or iatrogenic (damaged at the time of the pulmonary valve harvest), is probably the most obvious and also most disappointing exclusion to having the pulmonary autograft procedure.

TECHNICAL CONSIDERATIONS

In reviewing the technical operative goals of this procedure, one must examine three major areas as they relate to the intraoperative course of the procedure: (1) architecture of the transplanted pulmonary valve; (2) superior myocardial protection; and (3) perfect hemostasis. Success of this procedure is dependent on judicious focus and attention to these key details. Although efficient performance of this procedure intraoperatively is certainly paramount to the success of the pulmonary autograft procedure, the predominant operative goal should be a perfect anatomical result.

Architecture of the Transplanted Pulmonary Valve

The technique for insertion of the pulmonary autograft has changed since its inception in 1967. From 1967 to 1986, when the procedure was performed almost exclusively by Ross, the majority (90%) of all autografts were placed as subcoronary implants. The most recent Ross Registry data (1987 to the present) indicate that the trend is moving toward the root replacement (78%) implantation technique, which can be accomplished maintaining the relationships of the aortic valve complex. The subcoronary insertion technique accounts for 10% and the inclusion technique for the remaining 12% of the cases in the Registry.

Why this change in technique? The answer depends on several different variables. It is difficult, even in the most experienced hands, to maintain the precise architectural relationship inherent in the native aortic valve using the freehand scalloped subcoronary technique. On the other hand, this is easily within reach by using the root replacement technique, which requires the addition of the insertion of the coronary buttons into the pulmonary autograft.

Of the 20 autograft explants recorded in the current Registry data (2.0%), the early autograft explant rate is only 1.2% (10/820) with the root replacement technique, compared with 5.7% (6/105) with the subcoronary technique. The late results (5 to 15-year results) are not yet available, so to make a final decision in terms of implantation technique at this point would be premature.

The precise method for root insertion is still variable, especially in terms of running vs. interrupted suture techniques for the proximal suture line. This is also the case with the external reinforcement of the suture line with either Dacron, pericardium, or native aortic wall. There presently is no consensus or documented technique that clearly justifies one technique over the other. However, there is some agreement that some type of external annular support for the pulmonary autograft is beneficial in adults, whether the choice is Dacron or autologous pericardium. In infants and young children, in whom the growth potential of the autograft is at stake, any type of annular support would be counterproductive.

The root replacement techniques described herein are illustrated in Figures 2 through 4. Figure 2 illustrates the circular suture lines that allow accurate placement and correction of pulmonary-to-aortic annulus size discrepancy with interrupted suture lines proximally, and the preservation of sinotubular anatomy in the distal aortic suture line. Within the inset is the alternative of a running proximal suture line. Figure 3 illustrates the technique of external reinforcement using a supporting "ring" and interrupted sutures. Figure 4 demonstrates the completed operation with external annular support with emphasis on the placement of the left coronary button.

My preference for implantation of the aortic root is to use the entire pulmonary autograft as a root replacement as illustrated in Figure 2. The pulmonary autograft is then placed into the aortic annulus with interrupted sutures, with the use of external annular support in the form of autologous pericardium or Dacron as illustrated in Figure 3. Placement of individual interrupted sutures not only allows precise placement of sutures, but also achieves a staged plication of the aortic annulus or annuloplasty, thereby decreasing the likelihood of aortic annulus to pulmonary size mismatch. Leaflet coaptation is maximized using external annular support, thereby fixing the proximal suture line to the size of the pulmonary autograft. In addition, I prefer insertion of the aortic root before insertion of the pulmonary autograft because this allows for better visualization to secure hemostasis.

My choice of suture is 4–0 prolene with an RB-1 needle for proximal (interrupted) and distal (running) aortic and pulmonary suture lines. Either 5–0 or 6–0 prolene is used for the coronary ar-

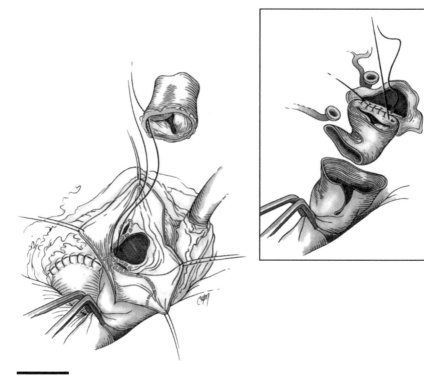

FIGURE 2.
Illustration of the circular suture lines allowing accurate placement and correction of pulmonary-to-aortic annulus size discrepancy with interrupted suture lines proximally and preservation of the sinotubular anatomy in the distal aortic suture line. **Inset,** demonstration of a running proximal suture line.

tery button anastomosis, with the opening in the autograft usually accomplished by a single longitudinal slit in the respective autograft sinus.

Optimal Myocardial Protection

The best method for achieving optimal myocardial protection is by means of a double venous cannulation with both vena cavae taped for complete diversion of blood. Systemic hypothermia (28° C to 32° C) allows for consistent moderate myocardial hypothermia with intermittent antegrade and retrograde cold blood cardioplegia. In the absence of uniform cardioplegia, topical cold saline is recommended because it provides anterior right ventricular cooling. To prevent phrenic nerve injury and attendant left ventricle warming, an insulating pad or jacket is mandated. Efficacy of these measures is guaranteed with continuous monitoring of the myocardial temperature during the intraoperative phase of the procedure. Optimum exposure and visualization as the pulmonary autograft is harvested and aortic root pathology is identified are achieved via left ventricular venting with either direct left ventricular apical venting or right superior pulmonary vein access. With these directives, the reconstruction of the aortic valve with the pulmonary autograft and the establishment of the RVOT with a pulmonary homograft, in mind, this technical procedure is well within the grasp of most surgeons.

Perfect Hemostasis

Adequate hemostasis intraoperatively is absolutely necessary for the success of the Ross procedure especially in lieu of the increased number of suture lines inherent in the pulmonary autograft procedure. The problem of inaccessible bleeding sites after bypass can be avoided by an exhaustive search for suture line bleeding while the aortic root is cold and the aortic root is pressurized. In addi-

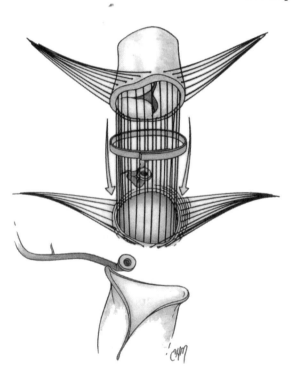

FIGURE 3.
Interrupted sutures plus supporting "ring."

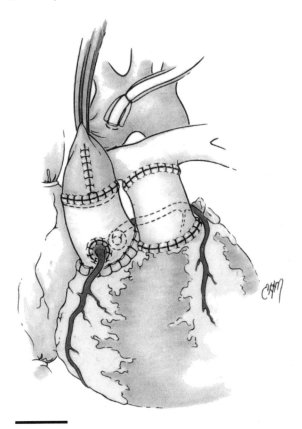

FIGURE 4.
Demonstration of the completed operation with external annular support.

tion, retrograde cardioplegia also facilitates the identification of venous sources of bleeding from the RVOT bed before placement of the pulmonary autograft for RVOT reconstruction.

CONCLUSION

The data available thus far in the Ross Registry confirm the efficacy of the Ross procedure as a solution for isolated aortic root pathology. The procedure can be achieved with a similar mortality rate to that of prosthetic valve replacement because of improved myocardial protection and an improved technical understanding of the procedure. The root replacement technique is evolving as the technique of choice for implantation. Technical variations continue to exist and are based primarily on each surgeon's operative philosophy. It would be optimal for all surgeons worldwide who are currently performing the Ross procedure to participate in the Ross Registry, because it is only through a worldwide cooperative effort that the long-term fate of the procedure can be evaluated.

REFERENCES

1. Czre LSC, Matloff JM, Chaux A, et al: The St. Jude valve: Analysis of thromboembolism, warfarin related hemorrhage and survival. *Am Heart J* 114:389–394, 1987.
2. Gallucci V, Bortolotti V, Milano, et al: The Hancock porcine valve 15 years later: An analysis of 575 patients, in Bodnar E, Yacoub M (eds): *Biologic and Bioprosthetic Valves*. New York, Yorke Medical Books, 1986, pp 91–97.
3. Schoen FJ, Levy RJ: Pathology of substitute heart valves: New concepts and developments. *J Card Surg* 9:222S–227S, 1994.
4. Lower RR, Stofer RC, Shumway NE: Autotransplantation of the pulmonic valve into the aorta. *J Thorac Cardiovasc Surg* 42:696–706, 1961.
5. Lower RR, Stofer RC, Shumway NE: Total excision of the mitral valve and replacement with the autologous pulmonary valve. *J Thorac Cardiovasc Surg* 42:696–706, 1961.
6. Pillsbury RC, Shumway NE: The replacement of the aortic valve with the autologous pulmonary valve. *Surgical Forum* 17:176–177, 1966.
7. Ross DN: Replacement of the aortic and pulmonary valves with the pulmonary autograft. *Lancet* 2:956–958, 1967.
8. Matsuki O, Okita Y, Almeida RS, et al: Two decades experience with aortic valve replacement with pulmonary autograft. *J Thorac Cardiovasc Surg* 95:705–711, 1988.
9. Gonzalez-Lavin L, Geens M, Ross D: Pulmonary valve autograft for aortic valve replacement. *J Thorac Cardiovasc Surg* 60:322, 1970.
10. Elkins RC, Santangelo KL, Randolph JD, et al: Pulmonary autograft replacement of the aortic valve: An evolution of technique. *J Card Surg* 7:108–116, 1992.
11. Elkins RC, Santangelo KL, Randolph JD, et al: Pulmonary autograft replacement in children: The ideal solution? *Ann Surg* 216:363–371, 1992.
12. Grunkemeier GL, Bodnar E: Comparative assessment of bioprosthetic durability in the aortic position. *J Heart Valve Dis* 4:49–55, 1995.
13. Ross D, Jackson M, Davies J: Pulmonary aortic valve replacement: Long term results. *J Card Surg* 6:529S–533S, 1991.
14. Stelzer P, Jones DJ, Elkin RC: Aortic root replacement with pulmonary autograft. *Circulation* 80:209–213, 1989.
15. Gorczynski A, Trenkner M, Anismomowicz L, et al: Biomechanics of the pulmonary valve in the aortic position. *Thorax* 37:535–539, 1982.
16. Iturbe-alessia J, Fonseca MDC, Mutchinik O, et al: Risks of anticoagulant therapy in pregnant women with artificial valves. *N Engl J Med* 315:1390–1393, 1986.

17. Agnihotri AK, McGiffin DC, Galbraith AJ, et al: The prevalence of infective endocarditis after aortic valve replacement. *J Thorac Cardiovasc Surg* 110:1708–1720, 1995.
18. Joyce F, Tingleff J, Pettersson G: The Ross operation in the treatment of prosthetic aortic valve endocarditis. *Semin Thorac Cardiovasc Surg* 7:38–46, 1995.
19. Oswalt JD, Dewan SJ: Aortic infective endocarditis managed by the Ross procedure. *J Heart Valve Dis* 2:380–384, 1993.
20. Oury JH, Eddy AC, Doty D, et al: Hemodynamic results of the Ross procedure in athletes. Presented at the Fourth Annual Ross Colloquium, 76th Annual Meeting of the AATS. San Diego, April 28, 1996.
21. Murata H: A study of autologous pulmonary valve replantation. *J Jpn Assoc Thorac Surg* 32:144–148, 1984.
22. Kumar N, Gallo R, Gometza B, et al: Pulmonary autograft for aortic valve disease: An ideal solution? *J Heart Valve Dis* 3:384–387, 1994.
23. Ross DN: Reflections on the pulmonary autograft (editorial). *J Heart Valve Dis* 2:363–364, 1993.

CHAPTER 3

Surgical Approach to Vascular Rings

Carl L. Backer, M.D.
Attending Surgeon, Division of Cardiovascular-Thoracic Surgery,
Children's Memorial Hospital; Associate Professor of Surgery,
Northwestern University Medical School, Chicago, Illinois

Constantine Mavroudis, M.D.
Head, Division of Cardiovascular-Thoracic Surgery, Children's Memorial
Hospital; Professor of Surgery, Northwestern University Medical School,
Chicago, Illinois

The phrase "vascular ring" was first used by Robert Gross in his report describing the first successful division of a double aortic arch in 1945.[1] Gross recalled his observations at the time of an autopsy performed in 1931 at which time he noted the anatomy of a 5-month-old infant who had died of vascular compression of the trachea.

> A ring of blood vessels was found encircling the intrathoracic portion of the esophagus and trachea in such a way that the esophagus was indented from behind, whereas the trachea was compressed on its anterior surface. The pathologic findings at once suggested that a division of some part of the so called "vascular ring" during life would probably have relieved the pressure on the constricted esophagus and trachea.[1]

Since that time, the phrase "vascular ring" has been used to refer to a group of congenital vascular anomalies that encircle and compress the esophagus and trachea. These infants usually have respiratory symptoms in the first few months of life and often require surgery within the first year of life.

The history of surgery for vascular rings began in 1945 when Gross[1] first divided a double aortic arch in a 1-year-old who had symptoms of wheezing respirations, cough, and recurrent tracheitis. Gross described the two classic vascular rings in that same monograph—right aortic arch with a left ligamentum and "divided

TABLE 1.
History of Vascular Ring Surgery

Year	Anomaly	Surgeon
1945	Double aortic arch	Robert E. Gross
1948	Innominate artery compression syndrome	Robert E. Gross
1954	Pulmonary artery sling	Willis J. Potts
1982	Complete tracheal rings	Farouk S. Idriss

aortic arch," now called double aortic arch. In 1948, Gross reported successful suspension of the innominate artery to the sternum for innominate artery compression syndrome in a 4-month-old infant with wheezing and respiratory distress.[2] In 1954, Willis J. Potts from Children's Memorial Hospital, Chicago, coined the term "pulmonary artery sling" in his report of successful repair of that anomaly in a 5-month-old with wheezing and intermittent attacks of dyspnea and cyanosis.[3] Finally, in 1982, Farouk S. Idriss from Children's Memorial Hospital reported the successful use of pericardium as a tracheoplasty technique for children with complete tracheal rings[4] (Table 1).

EMBRYOLOGY

The etiology of vascular rings is best understood by beginning with the embryonic aortic arches described by Congdon.[5] In the developing aortic arch system, there is both a ventral and a dorsal aorta, connected by the six primitive aortic arches (Fig 1). The first and second arches on either side contribute to minor facial arteries. The third arches become the carotid arteries. The development of the fourth arches determines whether a patient will have a normal left arch, a right arch, or a double aortic arch. The fifth arches bilaterally involute, and the dorsal portion of the left sixth arch becomes the patent ductus arteriosus. The ventral portion of the sixth arches becomes the proximal right and left pulmonary artery. The subclavian arteries develop from the seventh segmental arteries from the dorsal aorta.

This initial series of regressions and involutions develops first into the classic double aortic arch proposed by Edwards.[6] If the development of the arch is arrested at this stage, the vascular ring called a double aortic arch results. Normally, however, a portion of the right fourth arch and the right ductus involutes, leaving the patient with the normal left aortic arch and left-sided ductus arteriosus or ligamentum. By definition, a left aortic arch occurs when the apex of the aortic arch is to the left of the patient's trachea. In contrast, a right aortic arch is formed when the left fourth arch involutes and the right fourth arch persists. With this configuration, a number of different origins of the left subclavian artery and ligamentum arteriosum from the ascending and descending aorta can occur. When the left subclavian artery originates as the last arch vessel from the descending thoracic aorta and the ligamentum is from the main pulmonary artery to the descending thoracic aorta, a vascular ring is caused—the classic right aortic arch with left ligamentum arteriosum.

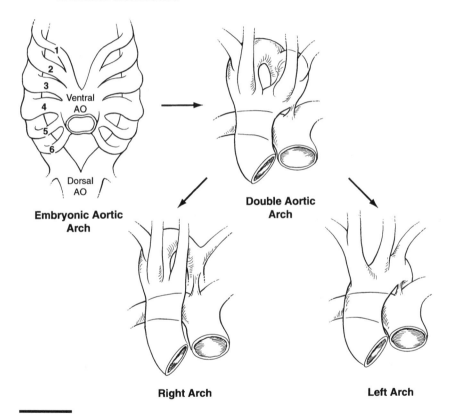

FIGURE 1.

In the embryonic aortic arch system the ventral and dorsal aorta *(AO)* are connected by six primitive aortic arches. The first, second, and fifth arches involute to form Edwards' classic double aortic arch. If the right fourth arch involutes, a normal left arch is formed. If the left fourth arch involutes, a right arch is formed.

TABLE 2.
Vascular Rings: Children's Memorial Hospital (1947–1996)

Anomaly	No. of Patients
Double aortic arch	88
Right aortic arch/left ligamentum	79
Innominate artery compression syndrome	81
Pulmonary artery sling	10
Complete tracheal rings	25
Ring-sling complex	10
Total	293

The embryologic etiology of innominate artery compression syndrome is thought to be abnormally posterior and leftward origination of the innominate artery from the ascending aorta. Pulmonary artery sling occurs when the developing left lung captures its arterial supply from derivatives of the *right* (instead of left) sixth aortic arch through capillaries *caudad* rather than cephalad to the developing tracheobronchial tree.[7] The embryologic etiology of complete tracheal rings is felt to be closely tied with pulmonary artery sling, both lesions being bronchopulmonary foregut malformations.[8]

CLINICAL PRESENTATION AND DIAGNOSIS

Between 1947 and 1996, 293 patients have undergone surgical repair of vascular rings or tracheal rings at the Children's Memorial Hospital in Chicago. Potts first reported division of a double aortic arch in 1948.[9] The institutional experience was summarized by Nikaidoh in 1972[10] (68 patients) and updated in 1989[11] (204 patients). Our current experience is shown in Table 2. Although there have been several different classification schemes proposed for vascular rings, we have preferred to simply call each vascular ring by its anatomical description rather than use a numbering or alphabetic lettering system.

Most infants with vascular rings have a combination of the following symptoms: stridor (noisy breathing), "seal-bark" cough, asthma, recurrent pneumonia, respiratory distress, cyanosis, dysphagia, and apnea. The true vascular rings, double aortic arch and right aortic arch with left ligamentum, often are associated with stridor and the "seal-bark" cough. This is particularly prominent and early in patients with a double aortic arch. Patients with pulmonary artery sling and complete tracheal rings often have respiratory distress, sometimes requiring emergent intubation and ventilation. Dysphagia tends to occur as a symptom only in older children who are taking solid foods. Infants with vascular rings who take formula do not have trouble swallowing in most cases. Apnea has been seen chiefly in patients with the innominate artery compression syndrome and complete tracheal rings.

Vascular rings are rare, and their diagnosis requires a heightened awareness for this diagnosis in any child with airway symptoms.[12] The diagnosis of vascular ring requires a sequential evaluation of the patient. Once the diagnosis has been obtained, it is important not to continue repeating examinations that simply reconfirm the diagnosis. Examinations that may lead to the correct diagnosis include (1) chest x-ray, (2) barium esophagram, (3) bronchoscopy, (4) echocardiogram, (5) CT/MRI, and (6) angiography.

The chest x-ray is useful in a number of ways. It can, in most cases, establish the location of the aortic arch. A right aortic arch should be visualized easily if this is present (Fig 2). In patients with a double aortic arch, it may be difficult to determine which side the arch is on, and this "indeterminate" arch location should make the physician consider double aortic arch as a diagnosis. The tracheal image on the chest x-ray in either case will show tracheal compression. In some cases, this can be highlighted by obtaining high-kV films of the airway. The chest x-ray can also be used to look for hyperinflation of the right lung that is often seen in patients with pulmonary artery sling. Patients with vascular rings may have areas of atelectasis or hyperinflation of other lobes related to compression from the ring. The chest x-ray in some cases has revealed a coin in the child's esophagus that has not passed because of the vascular ring.

The barium esophagram is the single most important and reliable technique for making the diagnosis of vascular ring.[13] It is also very cost-effective in the current era of managed care and capitation. The barium study will demonstrate compression of the esophagus by the vascular structures. In a patient with a double aortic arch, there will be compression from the right and left sides on the anteroposterior films and usually posteriorly on the lateral films (Fig 3). This compression is persistent in all views, which helps to differentiate this from a peristaltic wave. In patients with a right aortic arch and left ligamentum, there will be a prominent posterior and rightward compression from the right arch, indistinguishable from that shown in Figure 3. Pulmonary artery sling will cause anterior compression of the esophagus with no posterior component. The barium esophagram is essentially normal in a patient with innominate artery compression syndrome.

Bronchoscopy is used to evaluate a significant number of infants and young children with stridor.[14] Bronchoscopy of a patient with a vascular ring will demonstrate extrinsic compression of the trachea, which is easily dilated so that the scope can pass through. Bronchoscopy is used as the diagnostic procedure of choice for infants with complete tracheal rings. In patients with innominate artery compression syndrome, the trachea is compressed anteriorly by a pulsatile structure passing from left to right. Anterior posi-

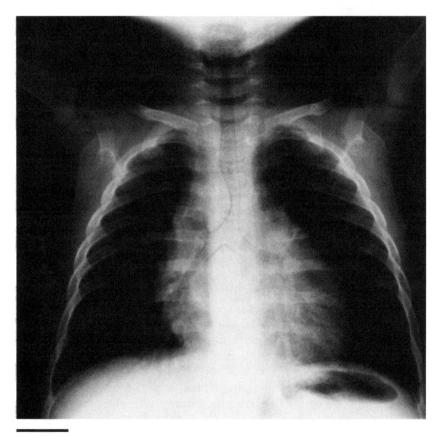

FIGURE 2.

Ten-month-old boy with stridor. Chest x-ray is significant for absence of left aortic knob. The tracheal air column has been highlighted to show the prominent right-sided compression of the trachea by a right aortic arch. The left side of the trachea is relatively straight.

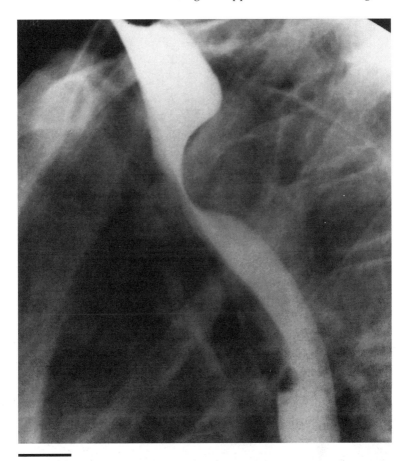

FIGURE 3.

Left lateral view of a double aortic arch as visualized on barium swallow in a 13-year-old boy. The prominent right arch is compressing the esophagus posteriorly.

tioning of the bronchoscope against the tracheal wall will obliterate the right radial pulse.

Echocardiography has recently become increasingly useful for the diagnosis of vascular rings.[15] The use of color-flow and Doppler interrogation has enhanced the sensitivity and specificity of echocardiography.[16] One limitation of echocardiography is that vascular ring segments without lumens cannot be visualized.[17] In our current practice, if a patient has complete tracheal rings diagnosed by bronchoscopy, we use echocardiography as the diagnostic procedure of choice to rule out pulmonary artery sling[18] (Fig

4). Echocardiography is also indicated to rule out a congenital heart lesion in a child with cyanotic spells.

Computed tomography and MRI are useful in that they identify both the vascular structures and the tracheobronchial anatomy.[19, 20] The CT scan, however, requires the administration of IV contrast material and exposes the child to radiation. Magnetic resonance imaging avoids these two issues but does require that the child be quite a bit more still during the procedure. In a child with an unstable airway, the MRI studies are sometimes not possible to obtain because of sedation concerns. These studies also have a high cost, which is a significant disadvantage. Figure 5, A demonstrates a CT scan, with contrast, of a child with double aortic arch. Figure 5, B, demonstrates the "four-vessel sign": in the superior mediastinum there are four brachiocephalic vessels identified separately, the right subclavian and carotid, and the left subclavian and carotid.[19] Patients with a right aortic arch also have the "four-vessel sign" (not shown).

Angiography was previously the diagnostic procedure of choice for vascular rings before the use of CT, MRI, and echocardi-

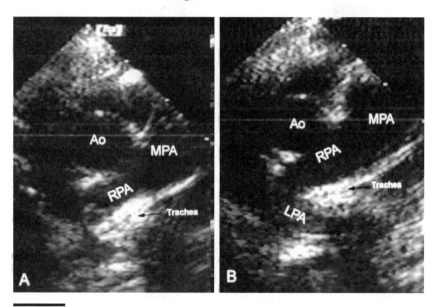

FIGURE 4.

Pulmonary artery sling as visualized on echocardiogram. Sequential sweeps **(A** and **B)** demonstrate the site of takeoff, course, and relative size of the left pulmonary artery *(LPA)* as it arises from the right pulmonary artery *(RPA)*. *Abbreviations: Ao,* aorta; *MPA,* main pulmonary artery.

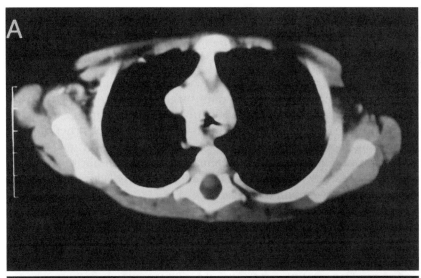

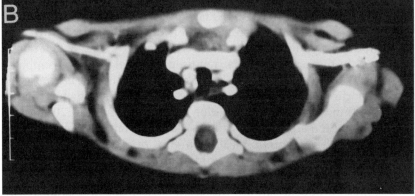

FIGURE 5.
A, computed tomography scan of a 13-month-old girl with "asthma" shows a double aortic arch. Trachea is compressed by the right and left arches. **B,** in the superior mediastinum the four-vessel sign is present. The brachiocephalic vessels are arranged symmetrically around the trachea posterior to the innominate vein.

ography.[21] However, in reality, the barium esophagram gives enough information in a child with stridor to have indications for surgical intervention. Although the barium esophagram does not necessarily reveal the precise diagnosis of the anatomy of the ring, it does reveal enough to know that the child has a vascular ring that requires division. For this reason, angiography is rarely, if ever, indicated except for very unusual cases or when the patient has an associated intracardiac defect that requires evaluation.

SURGICAL TECHNIQUES

Surgical intervention is indicated in all patients with clinical symptoms. Early and appropriate surgical repair helps avoid serious complications that can occur from hypoxic or apneic episodes. In addition, improper management of respiratory obstruction with prolonged intubation and nasogastric tube irritation may lead to catastrophic erosion of the trachea, esophagus, or aortic arch.[22–24] Other reported complications of an unrepaired vascular ring are aortic dissection and aneurysm.[25]

DOUBLE AORTIC ARCH

The double aortic arch (Table 3) typically causes the most severe and earliest onset of symptoms of the classic vascular rings. These infants frequently have the "seal-bark" type of chronic cough and nearly constant stridor. This is because the trachea is encircled by vascular structures that are all at aortic pressure and tightly configured. Two patients in our series were initially seen with a penny lodged in the esophagus that required removal with an esophagoscope. The most common form of double aortic arch is where the right aortic arch is dominant and the left arch is somewhat smaller (73%) (Fig 6). The left or anterior arch is dominant in 20% of patients, and the arches are equal in 7% of patients. A portion of the smaller arch was atretic in 30% to 40% of all cases. This area of atresia is usually at the insertion site of the lesser arch with the descending aorta. There is a separate origin of the right and left carotid and subclavian arteries from their respective arches with the carotid artery originating upstream to the subclavian.

The surgical approach to a double aortic arch is through a muscle-sparing left thoracotomy incision. The chest is entered through the fourth intercostal space. The pleura overlying the vascular ring should be opened and then careful dissection performed to identify clearly all the pertinent vascular structures, particularly the left subclavian artery, the ligamentum arteriosum, and the descending thoracic aorta. Then the left aortic arch should be clearly identified and mobilized. The right (posterior) arch does not require mobilization unless it is the smaller of the two arches. The lesser of the two arches should be divided at an appropriate point where the blood supply to the carotid and radial arteries is not affected. Gross originally described this as being between the left carotid and subclavian arteries. Since the double aortic arch was first

TABLE 3.
Summary of Diagnosis and Surgical Approach to Vascular Rings

Condition	Diagnostic Procedure of Choice	Surgical Approach	Procedure
Double Aortic Arch	Barium esophagram	Left thoracotomy	Divide lesser of two arches Divide ligamentum arteriosum Preserve blood flow to carotid/radial arteries
Right Aortic Arch/Left Ligamentum	Barium esophagram	Left thoracotomy	Divide ligamentum arteriosum Pex or resect Kommerell's diverticulum
Innominate Artery Compression Syndrome	Bronchoscopy	Right thoracotomy	Suspend innominate artery to posterior aspect of sternum
Pulmonary Artery Sling	Echocardiogram Bronchoscopy to rule out complete tracheal rings	Median sternotomy Cardiopulmonary bypass	Divide and oversew left pulmonary artery Implant left pulmonary artery into main pulmonary artery anterior to trachea
Complete Tracheal Rings	Bronchoscopy Echocardiography to rule out pulmonary artery sling	Median sternotomy Cardiopulmonary bypass	Tracheoplasty • Pericardial • Slide • Autograft • Resection with end-to-end anastomosis (short segment less than 1/3 trachea)

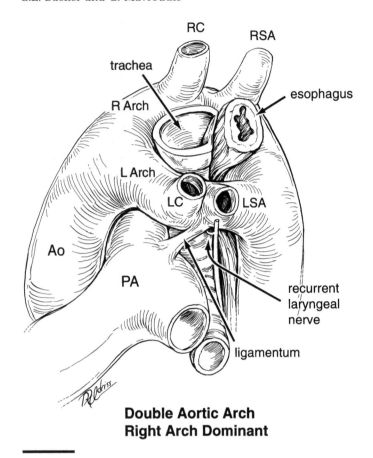

**Double Aortic Arch
Right Arch Dominant**

FIGURE 6.
Double aortic arch, right arch dominant. Left carotid artery *(LC)* and left subclavian artery *(LSA)* originate separately from the left aortic arch *(L Arch)*. *Abbreviations: Ao,* aorta; *PA,* pulmonary artery; *R Arch,* right aortic arch; *RC,* right carotid artery; *RSA,* right subclavian artery.

reported by Potts in 1948, we have usually selected as a site for arch division the place where the lesser arch inserts with the descending thoracic aorta. This area, as mentioned, is atretic in 30% to 40% of patients. Before dividing the arch, the arch should be temporarily occluded at the point that has been selected for division. Then the pulse in the right and left radial arteries, along with the right and left carotid arteries, should be checked by the anesthesiologist to ensure that the arch is not divided at a site that would interrupt blood flow to one of these vessels. This would be a potential problem if a portion of the arch that is atretic was left as the connecting arch to a brachiocephalic vessel. If the arches are similar in size, the distal blood pressure should also be checked to make sure it does not change. Arch division should be done between vascular clamps, either the Potts ductus clamps or the small Castaneda clamps (Fig 7). The ligamentum arteriosum should be divided or mobilized anteriorly with the arch division to prevent the ligamentum from combining with a persistent posterior right arch to make a loose vascular ring. The operative repair is completed by freeing up all adhesive bands surrounding the esophagus in the area of the divided arch. The mediastinal pleura is not sutured closed because this could contribute to scar formation that might recreate the problems caused by the original vascular ring.

One technical factor that the surgeon should be aware of is that when the clamps are placed on the vascular ring before ring division, the ring is temporarily tightened by inserting the clamps into the area between the ring and the trachea and esophagus. Patients at times will have a drop in their oxygen saturation and may require increased ventilatory pressures to provide adequate ventilation during the time that the clamps are on the vascular ring.

A possible pitfall in the surgical management of a child with a

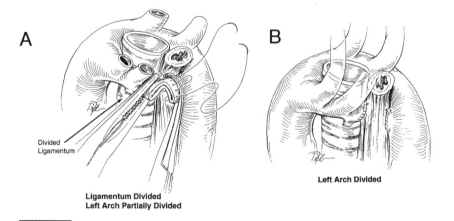

A

Divided
Ligamentum

**Ligamentum Divided
Left Arch Partially Divided**

B

Left Arch Divided

FIGURE 7.

A, exposure through a left thoracotomy incision. A patent left aortic arch is being divided. There is a Potts ductus clamp on the proximal portion of the arch and a Castaneda clamp on the distal arch adjacent to the descending thoracic aorta. The vascular ring has been partially transected with a single polypropylene suture placed on the distal portion of the divided arch. The ligamentum has already been divided and oversewn. **B,** completed repair with clamps removed. The stumps of the vascular rings have now separated approximately 2 cm.

double aortic arch occurs when the left arch is dominant and, at exploration through the left chest, initially no anomaly is noted. Only with careful dissection and inspection does one note that there can be a tiny right arch that is visible by reflecting the descending aorta anteriorly.

The postoperative care of the child after double aortic arch division involves monitoring in a high-acuity setting on the regular ward. Patients are kept under a high humidity head hood to loosen tracheobronchial secretions, and oxygen therapy is monitored with pulse oximetry. Some patients require chest physiotherapy and nasopharyngeal suctioning to encourage coughing and prevent atelectasis. Most patients will have a smoother postoperative course and shorter hospital stay if they are extubated immediately after the procedure. Noisy breathing will still be present in most patients immediately after the surgery. Sometimes this will be of such concern that the anesthesiologist considers reintubation of the child. Although the child has noisy breathing, this will usually not be significantly worse than before the surgery, and early extubation is preferable in nearly all instances. Complete relief of symptoms may not be noted immediately, and a period of months up to 1 year may pass before disappearance of noisy respirations. It is important that the parents be counseled as to this outcome before the surgery.

RIGHT AORTIC ARCH

Patients with a right aortic arch (see Table 3) generally are seen somewhat later in life than children with a double aortic arch because the ring is "looser," being formed partially by the low-pressure pulmonary artery and ligamentum arteriosum. Only older patients have dysphagia. One patient in our series was referred for diagnostic workup because he was always the last child at a meal to leave the table. He had learned that he needed to chew his food completely and carefully to swallow without discomfort. Chest x-ray demonstrates a right arch and compression of the right side of the trachea. Barium swallow in most instances confirms the diagnosis. There are two primary branching patterns of the brachiocephalic vessels in a patient with a right aortic arch: (1) retroesophageal left subclavian artery, and (2) mirror-image branching.[26] It is patients with retroesophageal left subclavian artery and a left ligamentum to the descending thoracic aorta who have a true vascular ring (Fig 8). When mirror-image branching is present, the ligamentum usually arises from the innominate artery and is anterior, so a complete vascular ring is not formed (Fig 9).

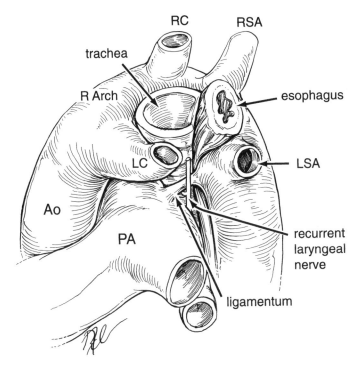

**Right Aortic Arch
Retroesophageal Left Subclavian Artery
Left Ligamentum**

FIGURE 8.
Illustration of right aortic arch *(R Arch)* with retroesophageal left subclavian artery *(LSA)* and left ligamentum arteriosum. The ring is formed by the right arch, pulmonary artery *(PA)*, and ligamentum. *Abbreviations: Ao,* aorta; *LC,* left carotid artery; *RC,* right carotid artery; *RSA,* right subclavian artery.

Frequently patients with a right aortic arch and left ligamentum will have a Kommerell's diverticulum develop at the origin of the left subclavian artery.[27] A Kommerell's diverticulum is a remnant of the left fourth arch. This diverticulum may enlarge and form an aneurysm that can compress surrounding structures (Fig 10). The Kommerell's diverticulum may not necessarily be diagnosed preoperatively by the barium swallow but should be looked for in all cases of right aortic arch with left ligamentum.

The surgical approach in a patient with right aortic arch and left ligamentum is through a muscle-sparing left thoracotomy in the fourth intercostal space. Dissection exposes the left subclavian artery, the ligamentum arteriosum, and the descending thoracic aorta. The phrenic, vagus, and recurrent laryngeal nerves are identified and protected. The ligamentum arteriosum is divided, using vascular clamps and staged division and oversewing of the stumps of the ligamentum arteriosum. This should clearly expose the esophagus, which is immediately beneath the ligamentum. Associated Kommerell's diverticulum should either be resected and oversewn with the use of a partial occlusion clamp or pexed to the adjacent

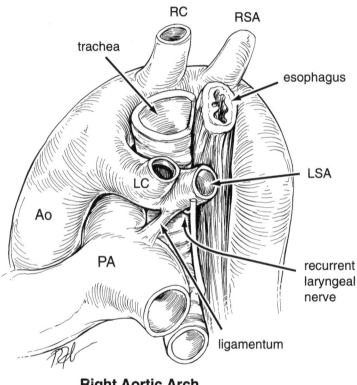

**Right Aortic Arch
Mirror Image Branching**

FIGURE 9.

In a right aortic arch with mirror-image branching, the ligamentum is often from the pulmonary artery *(PA)* to the left innominate artery and a complete vascular ring is *not* formed. *Abbreviations: Ao,* aorta; *LC,* left carotid artery; *LSA,* left subclavian artery; *RC,* right carotid artery; *RSA,* right subclavian artery.

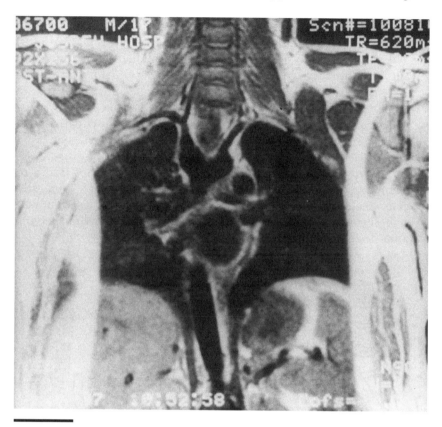

FIGURE 10.

An MRI scan showing aneurysm of Kommerell's diverticulum arising from descending aorta and serving as origin of left subclavian artery. (Courtesy of Backer CL, Ilbawi MN, Idriss FS, et al: Vascular anomalies causing tracheoesophageal compression: Review of experience in children. *J Thorac Cardiovasc Surg* 97:725–731, 1989.)

pleura or fascia of the vertebral column.[28] This prevents compression of the trachea or esophagus from the diverticulum itself. If ignored, this can be a source of residual postoperative symptoms. Any adhesive bands crossing over the esophagus should be divided.

Some surgeons have recommended ligating and dividing the left subclavian artery in addition to the ligamentum to achieve relief of vascular compression in patients with a right aortic arch.[29] In our experience, we have not found this to be necessary. An unusual group of patients with a right aortic arch and left ligamentum have a left-sided descending aorta, the so-called circumflex aorta (Fig 11, left). Robotin and associates have described an aortic "uncrossing" operation for these rare patients[30] (3 of 468 patients). This procedure is performed through a median sternotomy with cardiopulmonary bypass and hypothermic circulatory arrest. The aortic arch is mobilized, divided, and brought in front of the tracheobronchial tree, then reanastomosed end-to-side to the lateral aspect of the ascending aorta (Fig 11, right). All three patients described by Robotin had prior ligamentum division via left thoracotomy. Although 30% of patients with truncus arteriosus and tetralogy of Fallot have a right aortic arch,[31] we did not find a reverse association with a specific cardiac defect when a vascular ring was formed by a right arch. Postoperative care of a patient with right aortic arch and left ligamentum is similar to that for patients after double aortic arch division.

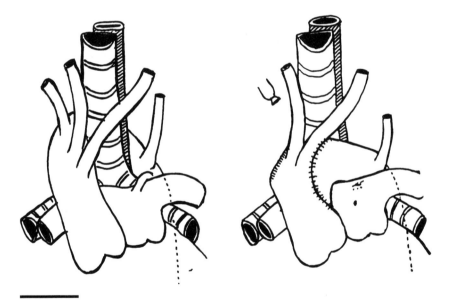

FIGURE 11.

Left, anatomy of a child with a "circumflex aorta." A right-sided aortic arch passes over the right main bronchus, then takes a retroesophageal course and joins the left-sided descending aorta. **Right,** aortic uncrossing procedure completed. The right subclavian artery has been ligated and divided. The aortic arch was transected proximal to the origin of the right subclavian artery, mobilized, and reanastomosed to the left side of the ascending aorta and left carotid artery in front of the trachea. (Courtesy of Robotin MC, Bruniaux J, Serraf A, et al: Unusual forms of tracheobronchial compression in infants with congenital heart disease. *J Thorac Cardiovasc Surg* 112:415–423, 1996.)

INNOMINATE ARTERY COMPRESSION SYNDROME

Innominate artery compression of the trachea (see Table 3) in infants can cause stridor, cyanosis, apnea, and respiratory arrest. These episodes have been referred to as "dying spells." Frequently this apnea is associated with swallowing a bolus of food. The pathophysiology is felt to be a reflex apnea caused by a combination of anterior compression of the trachea by the innominate artery and then posterior compression of the membranous portion of the trachea by the bolus of food passing through the esophagus. These patients also have stridor and can have recurrent upper respiratory tract infections. They may also have a characteristic posture with opisthotonos and hyperextension of the head.[2]

The diagnosis of innominate artery compression syndrome is made by rigid bronchoscopy. Bronchoscopy demonstrates an anterior compression of the trachea that progresses from less severe on the left side to most severe on the right side. Some narrowing of the airway from the innominate artery can be seen in patients without symptoms, and we have used a criterion of 75% narrowing before considering patients for surgical intervention. This compression is pulsatile and is easily opened by the tip of the rigid bronchoscope. Lifting the bronchoscope anteriorly causes obliteration of the right radial pulse because of the compression of the innominate artery. The innominate artery compression syndrome can be confirmed by CT with administration of contrast material (Fig 12).

Our approach to repair of innominate artery compression syndrome is similar to that originally reported by Gross in 1948,[2] with the exception that Gross approached his patient through a left thoracotomy and we have performed this operation through a right thoracotomy. The thoracotomy is an anterolateral thoracotomy performed through the third intercostal space anteriorly. The right lobe of the thymus is resected, with care taken to preserve the phrenic nerve. This allows access to the area of the superior mediastinum where the pericardium is opened to identify the innominate artery originating from the aorta. Three separate polypropylene sutures, all buttressed with felt pledgets, are passed through the innominate artery. These sutures go through the adventitia of the vessel without entering the actual vessel lumen. One is placed on the innominate artery, one placed through the pericardial junction or reflection with the innominate artery, and the last placed on the ascending aorta just at the base of the innominate artery. These three sutures are then passed through the posterior table of the sternum and then tied. This elevates the anterior tracheal wall and opens the tracheal lumen, as is illustrated in Figure 13.

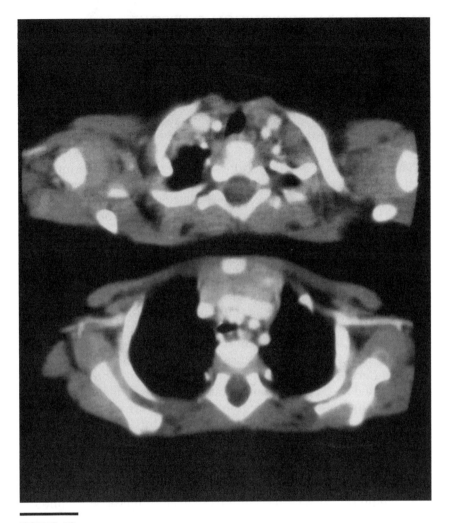

FIGURE 12.
Computed tomography scan demonstrating innominate artery compression syndrome. In the **upper panel,** the normal tracheal lumen is seen. In the **lower panel,** the trachea is compressed by the innominate artery. (Courtesy of Backer CL, Mavroudis C: Vascular rings and pulmonary artery sling, in Mavroudis C, Backer CL (eds): *Pediatric Cardiac Surgery,* ed 2. St. Louis, Mosby, 1994, p 155.)

Recently, Hawkins and colleagues reported treatment of patients with innominate artery compression syndrome using a median sternotomy approach with division and reimplantation of the innominate artery into the aorta at a site to the right of the original takeoff.[32] This technique not only requires a median sternotomy but carries the additional risk of bleeding, stroke, and anastomotic stricture.[33] It also sacrifices the active suspending mechanism of pulling the anterior tracheal wall open that is achieved in innominate arteriopexy.[34] Other centers have also reported excellent results with innominate arteriopexy.[33, 35, 36]

ABERRANT RIGHT SUBCLAVIAN ARTERY

Left aortic arch with aberrant right subclavian artery occurring as the last brachiocephalic branch from the descending aorta is the

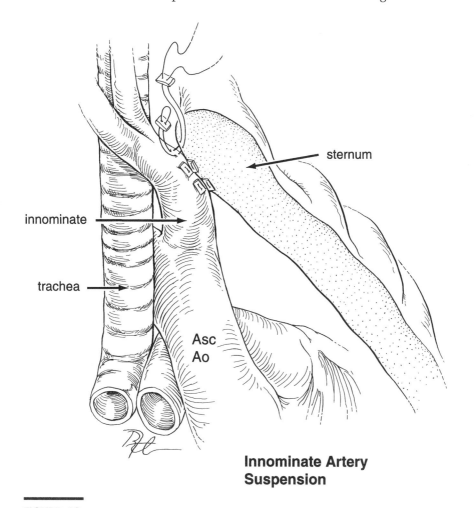

Innominate Artery Suspension

FIGURE 13.

Fixing the adventitia of the innominate artery to the posterior table of the sternum with pledgetted sutures pulls the innominate artery anteriorly and actively pulls the tracheal wall forward and opens it. *Abbreviation: Asc Ao,* ascending aorta.

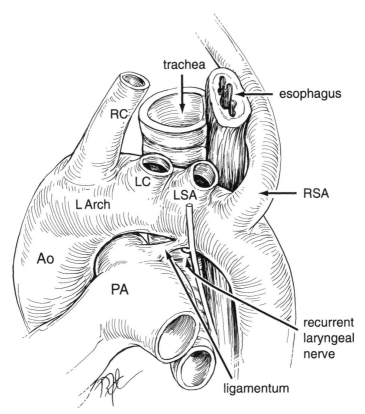

**Left Aortic Arch
Aberrant Right Subclavian Artery**

FIGURE 14.

Left aortic arch *(L Arch)* with aberrant origin of the right subclavian artery *(RSA)* as the last brachiocephalic vessel from the aortic arch. *Abbreviations: Ao,* aorta; *LC,* left carotid artery; *LSA,* left subclavian artery; *PA,* pulmonary artery; *RC,* right carotid artery.

most common vascular anomaly of the aortic arch system (0.5%).[37] This produces a posterior indentation of the esophagus on barium swallow, but does not form a complete vascular ring (Fig 14). Because it is so common, in the past it was often blamed for a child's vague symptoms, which then persisted after ligation and division of the right subclavian artery. This earned the lesion the name, "dysphagia lusoria,"[38] meaning "trick of nature." The aberrant right subclavian is a "red herring" that is almost always *not* the etiology of the child's symptoms.[39] At Children's Memorial Hospital, seven patients had ligation of an aberrant right subclavian artery through a left thoracotomy, all before 1973. These patients are not included in Table 2 because we no longer consider the lesion to be a type of vascular ring. It should be noted that in adults, the base of the aberrant right subclavian artery may become dilated and aneurysmal, compressing the esophagus and causing dysphagia. If this occurs, the aneurysm should be resected and the right subclavian artery divided and implanted into the aorta or right carotid artery. This has been accomplished through both left[40] and right[41] thoracotomy approaches.

PULMONARY ARTERY SLING

A pulmonary artery sling (see Table 3) is formed when the left pulmonary artery originates from the right pulmonary artery and encircles the distal trachea and right mainstem bronchus, and courses between the trachea and the esophagus to the left lung (Fig 15). The left pulmonary artery acts as a sling that applies pressure on the right mainstem bronchus and lower trachea, causing tracheobronchial malacia and stenosis at these sites. This anomaly was first reported by Glaevecke and Doehle (in 1897) as an autopsy finding in a 7-month-old infant who had had severe respiratory distress.[42] Nearly all infants with this diagnosis are seen within the first few months of life with respiratory distress. The chest radiograph may show unilateral hyperinflation of the right lung. Barium esophagram shows anterior compression of the esophagus on lateral views: this relationship is demonstrated in the inset for Figure 15. Echocardiography is our diagnostic procedure of choice for pulmonary artery sling.[18] Two-dimensional color Doppler echocardiogram, using suprasternal/high parasternal sweeps, diagnosed pulmonary artery sling in 7 of 7 patients (100%) (see Fig 4). Both CT and MRI will also show the left pulmonary artery originating from the right pulmonary artery and encircling the trachea. Bronchoscopy should be performed in all infants with diagnosed pulmonary artery sling to evaluate for associated complete tracheal rings. In our series of 20 patients with pulmonary artery sling, 10 (50%) had associated complete tracheal rings. Berdon and colleagues have appropriately referred to this as the "ring-sling complex."[43]

Surgical repair of pulmonary artery sling should be undertaken as soon as the diagnosis is made because of the tenuous nature of the respiratory status of the child. The first successful operation for a pulmonary artery sling was performed by Dr. Willis Potts at Children's Memorial Hospital in 1954 through a right thoracotomy.[3]

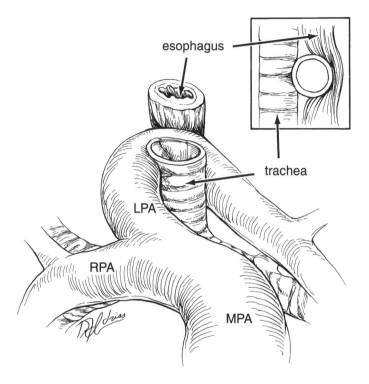

Pulmonary Artery Sling

FIGURE 15.

Pulmonary artery sling. The left pulmonary artery *(LPA)* originates from the right pulmonary artery *(RPA)* and courses between the esophagus and trachea to reach the left lung. *Inset* shows lateral relationship of LPA to esophagus. It is this view that can be diagnostic on a barium swallow. *Abbreviation: MPA,* main pulmonary artery.

Potts operated on a 5-month-old infant who did not have an exact preoperative diagnosis but was felt to have vascular compression of the lower trachea and right bronchus by a vascular structure of some sort. He made the correct intraoperative diagnosis and considered several surgical alternatives, including right pneumonectomy, before deciding to transect the left pulmonary artery and reanastomose it to the main pulmonary artery anterior to the trachea. That particular child survived the surgery and is still alive; however, the left pulmonary artery is occluded.[44] The second patient in our series was operated on through a median sternotomy without cardiopulmonary bypass and survived, but also has an occluded left pulmonary artery. Occlusion of the left pulmonary artery after pulmonary artery sling repair continued to be a problem in several other surgical series.[7, 45] The next six patients undergoing operations at Children's Memorial Hospital were approached through a left thoracotomy.[46]

In 1985, the first patient to undergo simultaneous repair of pulmonary artery sling and complete tracheal rings at Children's Memorial Hospital was operated on through a median sternotomy approach. Since that time, all patients with pulmonary artery sling have been approached through a median sternotomy whether or not they have associated complete tracheal rings.[47] Median sternotomy is performed and the child is placed on cardiopulmonary bypass with aortic cannulation and single right atrial cannulation. The child is cooled to 32°C slowly so that the heart remains in normal sinus rhythm throughout the procedure. The left pulmonary artery is identified originating from the posterior aspect of the right pulmonary artery, just to the right of the trachea. The left pulmonary artery is dissected into the posterior mediastinum as far as possible from the right side. This dissection should proceed cautiously, particularly in relationship to the membranous portion of the trachea posteriorly, which can be inadvertently entered if these structures are densely adherent. The pericardium is opened at the left posterior aspect of the pericardial sac at a site just inferior to where the ligamentum attaches to the descending thoracic aorta. It is in this area that the left pulmonary artery can be identified beneath the pericardium but anterior to the aorta where it courses into the left hilum. The right pulmonary artery is partially occluded with a vascular clamp, and the left pulmonary artery is transected from its origin from the right pulmonary artery. The resultant opening in the right pulmonary artery is closed with interrupted polypropylene sutures. The transected left pulmonary artery is then passed through the mediastinum posterior to the trachea and brought up through the opening in the pericardium created on the left side. A partial occlusion clamp is then placed on the main pulmonary artery in a posterior site, selected to give the left pulmonary artery a natural "lie." The left pulmonary artery is anastomosed to the main pulmonary artery using interrupted polypropylene or polydioxanone suture. The completed repair is illustrated in Figure 16.

An alternative technique for repair of pulmonary artery sling was described by Jonas.[48] This approach involved transecting the trachea, resecting the stenotic portion of the trachea, relocating the left pulmonary artery anterior to the trachea, and then anastomosing the trachea back together. This relieves the sling-type effect of the pulmonary artery on the distal trachea and right mainstem bronchus without a vascular anastomosis. However, it does not correct the abnormal rightward takeoff of the left pulmonary artery from the main pulmonary artery, leading to possible kinking of the left pulmonary artery. Although we have preferred a median sternotomy approach with cardiopulmonary bypass for pulmonary artery sling repair, it should be noted that Pawade and associates described 14 of 18 patients who had a patent left pulmonary artery after repair via left thoracotomy.[49]

The Children's Memorial Hospital experience with pulmonary artery sling has involved 20 infants with a mean age of 4 months at the time of surgery. Ten patients had associated complete tracheal rings—the "ring-sling complex." There has been no operative mortality in these patients. There were two late deaths for a 10% overall mortality. Both were patients with associated complete tracheal rings having simultaneous tracheoplasty. The patency rate of the left pulmonary artery using a median sternotomy and cardiopulmonary bypass is 100%, and the mean blood flow to the left lung in our series by nuclear scan is 42.7%.

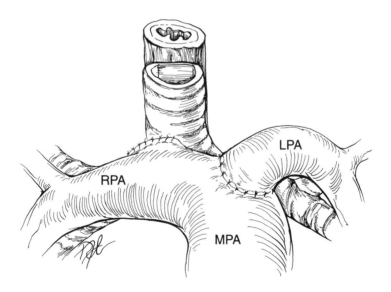

Repaired Pulmonary Artery Sling

FIGURE 16.
Completed repair of pulmonary artery sling. *Abbreviations: RPA*, right pulmonary artery; *LPA*, left pulmonary artery; *MPA*, main pulmonary artery.

COMPLETE TRACHEAL RINGS

Complete tracheal rings (see Table 3) occur when there is congenital absence of the membranous trachea (Fig 17). This causes severe tracheal stenosis leading to respiratory distress in infancy. Benjamin reported that the medical management of this lesion is associated with a 43% mortality rate.[50] Other authors have reported a similar high mortality rate from complete tracheal rings.[51] Although the number of the rings and extent of the stenosis can be variable, most of our patients have had complete tracheal rings from one or two rings below the cricoid extending to the carina. Cantrell and Guild[52] categorized complete tracheal rings into three categories: segmental stenosis, funnel-like stenosis, and generalized hypoplasia. The diagnosis of complete tracheal rings is by rigid bronchoscopy. The bronchoscope is used to demonstrate the absence of a membranous septum and presence of complete circumferential cartilaginous rings. In many of these patients, the bronchoscope itself cannot be passed through the stenosis, but only the fine telescope. All patients with diagnosed complete tracheal rings should have a pulmonary artery sling ruled out by evaluating the patient with an echocardiogram or, if the child is taken urgently to surgery, by direct intraoperative inspection.

Surgical options described for patients with complete tracheal rings include pericardial patch tracheoplasty,[4, 53] resection with end-to-end anastomosis,[54] cartilage tracheoplasty,[55] and slide tracheoplasty.[56, 57] At the Children's Memorial Hospital from 1982 to 1996, 28 patients have undergone pericardial tracheoplasty,[58, 59] 2 patients have undergone slide tracheoplasty,[60] 2 have had resection of short segments of complete rings, and 3 patients have undergone a tracheal autograft technique.[61] Ten patients (29%) had simultaneous pulmonary artery sling repair. Five patients (14%) had simultaneous intracardiac repair of atrioventricular canal, double-outlet right ventricle, tetralogy of Fallot, ventricular septal defect with pulmonary artery sling, and pulmonary atresia. Six patients (17%) had an associated tracheal right upper lobe bronchus.

The technique for tracheoplasty uses a median sternotomy approach and cardiopulmonary bypass for respiratory support. Bronchoscopic guidance for an anterior incision in the trachea is used for pericardial patch tracheoplasty. The trachea is patched with an autologous pericardial patch anchored with interrupted 6–0 Vicryl sutures (Fig 18). The patch is typically 1.5–2.0 cm in width and extends for the length of the tracheal stenosis, usually 3.0–5.0 cm. The patch is stented with an endotracheal tube for 7–10 days, at which time the child is weaned from the ventilator and extubated.

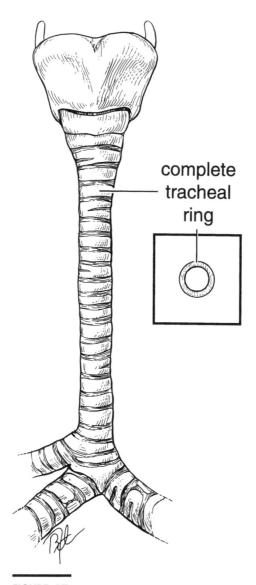

complete
tracheal
ring

FIGURE 17.
Complete tracheal rings causing long-segment congenital tracheal stenosis from the third tracheal ring to the carina. This patient has an associated tracheal right upper lobe bronchus.

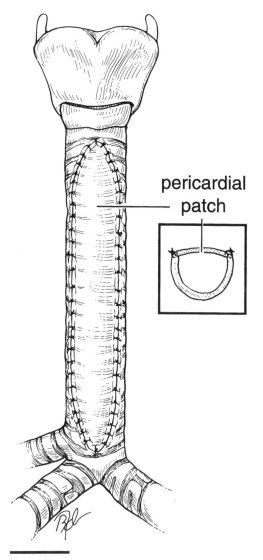

FIGURE 18.
Completed pericardial patch tracheoplasty augments the trachea anteriorly, opening the tracheal lumen significantly as shown in the *inset.*

Bronchoscopy is performed before extubation to remove secretions and granulation tissue, and perform dilation if necessary.[59]

We have used the pericardial patch technique in 28 patients, with 2 early and 4 late deaths. Twenty-two patients (78%) are alive and doing well. One early death was from patch dehiscence and mediastinitis, and the other was related to postoperative extracorporeal membrane oxygenation complications. Three late deaths were related to residual airway stenosis, and one to pulmonary hypertension (Down's syndrome with atrioventricular canal). Six patients had surgical revision of their tracheoplasty, four with autologous costal cartilage grafts and two with autologous pericardium.[62] Three patients have had placement of balloon expandable metallic Palmaz stents for collapsing tracheal or bronchial segments.[63] These stents were placed into the distal trachea and/or proximal bronchi during bronchoscopy with fluoroscopic guidance. In each case, the patency of the lumen was successfully maintained without promoting excessive granulation tissue.

The slide tracheoplasty was first described by Tsang and Goldstraw[56] and was recently modified by Grillo.[57] We have used this technique with a median sternotomy approach and the use of cardiopulmonary bypass. The mid-portion of the trachea is identified bronchoscopically. Then the trachea is transected at this site. The lower trachea is opened anteriorly, the upper trachea is opened posteriorly. The two tracheal openings then "slide," one on top of the other, trimming the very corners of the transected trachea. The two are anastomosed with interrupted Vicryl sutures. This creates a trachea that is one-half as long as the original but has four times the diameter. Of course, the patient still has complete circumferential tracheal rings. We have used this technique in two infants.[61] One child did very well and was discharged at 18 days; the other had considerable growth of granulation tissue and tracheomalacia requiring a stent, and eventually died four months postoperatively.

The autograft technique (median sternotomy, cardiopulmonary bypass) involves incising the trachea anteriorly throughout the length of the stenosis. Then approximately six rings or 15 mm of trachea are harvested from the mid-portion of the trachea. The trachea is reanastomosed posteriorly with interrupted 6–0 Vicryl suture. The autograft is used as a distal patch at the critical junction of the carina and left and right mainstem bronchus. In patients with a short segment of stenosis, the autograft acts to complete the tracheal patch anteriorly. In patients with longer stenosis, this has been augmented superiorly with pericardium. We have used this technique successfully in three infants, one with associated ventricular septal defect and pulmonary artery sling, one with associated pulmonary artery sling, and one with Down's syndrome.

VIDEO-ASSISTED THORACOSCOPIC SURGERY

There have recently been reports of using video-assisted thoracoscopic surgery (VATS) for the division of vascular rings.[64] This has occurred as an extension of the use of VATS for patent ductus arteriosus ligation.[65] Burke[66] reported the use of VATS for eight patients with vascular rings. Anatomy of the rings included double aortic arch with an atretic left arch (3 patients) and right aortic arch, left ligamentum arteriosum (5 patients). Three patients (37.5%) required a thoracotomy to complete the procedure. The median operating time was 4 hours, and the median hospital stay was 3 days. It is interesting to note there were no patients with a patent arch. A real concern for the patient with a patent arch is that once the clips are applied and the ring divided, the two stumps retract because of the tension on the ring. The posterior stump often retracts into the mediastinum, and if the clip should slip off, the risk of hemorrhage is great. It is not always possible to tell externally whether a segment of the ring is atretic or patent.

RARE VASCULAR RINGS

There are several highly unusual types of vascular rings for which there are only isolated case reports in the literature. In fact, none of the lesions described in this section have been diagnosed in our series of nearly 300 patients at Children's Memorial Hospital. The first of these is the left aortic arch, right descending aorta, and right ligamentum arteriosum.[67] The left arch in these cases is often a cervical arch resulting from the arch developing from the third rather than fourth left arch.[68] These patients frequently have associated cardiac anomalies such as absent left pulmonary artery, ventricular septal defect, tetralogy of Fallot, and transposition of the great arteries.[69] Approximately 19 of these cases have been reported in the world literature.[70] This is one of the very rare lesions best approached with a right thoracotomy[71] rather than a left thoracotomy. Because of the associated cardiac anomalies, these patients usually will have an extensive evaluation including cardiac catheterization and echocardiogram. The appearance on esophagram is very distinctive and should raise a "red flag" for further evaluation before surgical intervention.[72]

Binet[73] reported a single case of a ductus arteriosus connecting the right pulmonary artery to the descending aorta between the trachea and esophagus with an aberrant right subclavian artery. Ben-Shachar[74] reported a hemitruncal sling creating a vascular ring. The right pulmonary artery originated from the ascending aorta and coursed in a dorsocranial direction wrapping around the trachea.

CONCLUSION

Vascular rings are rare congenital anomalies that cause compression of the trachea and esophagus. Infants can have stridor, cyanosis, respiratory distress, and apnea. Diagnosis is best established by esophagram for double aortic arch and right aortic arch with left ligamentum. Bronchoscopy is used to diagnose innominate artery compression syndrome and complete tracheal rings. Echocardiogram is the diagnostic procedure of choice for pulmonary artery sling. The surgical approaches to vascular rings include a left thoracotomy for double aortic arch and right aortic arch with left ligamentum, right thoracotomy for innominate artery suspension, and median sternotomy with extracorporeal circulation for pulmonary artery sling and complete tracheal rings. There has been no operative mortality from an isolated vascular ring or pulmonary artery sling at Children's Memorial Hospital since 1959. The survival rate of infants with complete tracheal rings in our series is 83%, and mortality has been related to residual airway stenosis. Ninety-two percent of all infants who undergo vascular ring repair are free of respiratory symptoms at 1 year postoperatively.

REFERENCES

1. Gross RE: Surgical relief for tracheal obstruction from a vascular ring. *N Engl J Med* 233:586–590, 1945.
2. Gross RE, Neuhauser EBD: Compression of the trachea by an anomalous innominate artery: An operation for its relief. *Am J Dis Child* 75:570–574, 1948.
3. Potts WJ, Holinger PH, Rosenblum AH: Anomalous left pulmonary artery causing obstruction to right main bronchus: Report of a case. *JAMA* 155:1409–1411, 1954.
4. Idriss FS, DeLeon SY, Ilbawi MN, et al: Tracheoplasty with pericardial patch for extensive tracheal stenosis in infants and children. *J Thorac Cardiovasc Surg* 88:527–536, 1984.
5. Congdon ED: Transformation of the aortic arch system during the development of the human embryo. *Contrib Embryol* 14:47–110, 1992.
6. Edwards JE: Anomalies of derivatives of aortic arch system. *Med Clin North Am* 32:925–949, 1948.
7. Sade RM, Rosenthal A, Fellows K, et al: Pulmonary artery sling. *J Thorac Cardiovasc Surg* 69:333–346, 1975.
8. Rodgers BM, Harman PK, Johnson AM: Bronchopulmonary foregut malformations. *Ann Surg* 203:517–524, 1986.
9. Potts WJ, Gibson S, Rothwell R: Double aortic arch: Report of two cases. *Arch Surg* 57:227–233, 1948.
10. Nikaidoh H, Riker WL, Idriss FS: Surgical management of "vascular rings." *Arch Surg* 105:327–333, 1972.
11. Backer CL, Ilbawi MN, Idriss FS, et al: Vascular anomalies causing tracheoesophageal compression: Review of experience in children. *J Thorac Cardiovasc Surg* 97:725–731, 1989.
12. Lowe GM, Donaldson JS, Backer CL: Vascular rings: 10-year review of imaging. *Radiographics* 11:637–646, 1991.

13. Stark J, Roesler M, Chrispin A, et al: The diagnosis of airway obstruction in children. *J Pediatr Surg* 20:113–117, 1985.
14. Holinger LD: Diagnostic endoscopy of the pediatric airway. *Laryngoscope* 99:346–348, 1989.
15. Chin AJ, Fogel MA: *Noninvasive Imaging of Congenital Heart Disease: Before and After Surgical Reconstruction.* Armonk, NY, Futura, 1994, pp 216–218.
16. Alboliras ET, Lombardo S, Antillon J: Truncus arteriosus with double aortic arch: Two-dimensional and color flow Doppler echocardiographic diagnosis. *Am Heart J* 129:415–417, 1995.
17. Murdison KA, Andrews BAA, Chin AJ: Ultrasonographic display of complex vascular rings. *J Am Coll Cardiol* 15:1645–1653, 1990.
18. Alboliras ET, Backer CL, Holinger LD, et al: Pulmonary artery sling: Diagnostic and management strategy. *Pediatrics* 98:530A, 1996.
19. McLoughlin MJ, Weisbrod G, Wise DJ, et al: Computed tomography in congenital anomalies of the aortic arch and great vessels. *Radiology* 138:399–403, 1981.
20. Julsrud PR, Ehman RL: Magnetic resonance imaging of vascular rings. *Mayo Clin Proc* 61:181–185, 1986.
21. Azarow KS, Pearl RH, Hoffman MA, et al: Vascular ring: Does magnetic resonance imaging replace angiography? *Ann Thorac Surg* 53:882–885, 1992.
22. Arciniegas E, Hakimi M, Hertzler JH, et al: Surgical management of congenital vascular rings. *J Thorac Cardiovasc Surg* 77:721–727, 1979.
23. Othersen HB Jr, Khalil B, Zellner J, et al: Aortoesophageal fistula and double aortic arch: Two important points in management. *J Pediatr Surg* 31:594–595, 1996.
24. Heck HA Jr, Moore HV, Lutin WA, et al: Esophageal-aortic erosion associated with double aortic arch and tracheomalacia: Experience with 2 infants. *Tex Heart Inst J* 20:126–129, 1993.
25. Midulla PS, Dapunt OE, Sadeghi AM, et al: Aortic dissection involving a double aortic arch with a right descending aorta. *Ann Thorac Surg* 58:874–875, 1994.
26. Felson B, Palayew MJ: The two types of right aortic arch. *Radiology* 81:745–759, 1963.
27. Kommerell B: Verlagerung des osophagus durch eine abnorm verlaufende arteria subclavia dextra (arteria lusoria). *Fortschr Geb Rontgenstr* 54:590, 1936.
28. Chun K, Colombani PM, Dudgeon DL, et al: Diagnosis and management of congenital vascular rings: A 22-year experience. *Ann Thorac Surg* 53:597–602, 1992.
29. Jung JY, Almond CH, Saab SB, et al: Surgical repair of right aortic arch with aberrant left subclavian artery and left ligamentum arteriosum. *J Thorac Cardiovasc Surg* 75:237–243, 1978.
30. Robotin MC, Bruniaux J, Serraf A, et al: Unusual forms of tracheobronchial compression in infants with congenital heart disease. *J Thorac Cardiovasc Surg* 112:415–423, 1996.
31. Hastreiter AR, D'Cruz IA, Cantez T, et al: Right-sided aorta: I. Occur-

rence of right aortic arch in various types of congenital heart disease. II. Right aortic arch, right descending aorta, and associated anomalies. *Br Heart J* 28:722–739, 1966.

32. Hawkins JA, Bailey WW, Clark SM: Innominate artery compression of the trachea. Treatment by reimplantation of the innominate artery. *J Thorac Cardiovasc Surg* 103:678–682, 1992.

33. Adler SC, Isaacson G, Balsara RK: Innominate artery compression of the trachea: Diagnosis and treatment by anterior suspension. A 25-year experience. *Ann Otol Rhinol Laryngol* 104:924–927, 1995.

34. Backer CL, Holinger LD, Mavroudis C: Innominate artery compression: Division and reimplantation versus suspension [Invited letter and commentary]. *J Thorac Cardiovasc Surg* 103:817–820, 1992.

35. Jones DT, Jonas RA, Healy GB: Innominate artery compression of the trachea in infants. *Ann Otol Rhinol Laryngol* 103:347–350, 1994.

36. Moes CAF, Izukawa T, Trusler GA: Innominate artery compression of the trachea. *Arch Otolaryngol* 101:733–738, 1975.

37. Abbott ME: *Atlas of Congenital Heart Disease.* New York, American Heart Association, 1936.

38. Gross RE: Surgical treatment for dysphagia lusoria. *Ann Surg* 124:532–534, 1946.

39. Beabout JW, Stewart JR, Kincaid OW: Aberrant right subclavian artery, dispute of commonly accepted concepts. *Am J Roentgen* 92:855–864, 1964.

40. Pifarre R, Dieter RA Jr, Niedballa RG: Definitive surgical treatment of the aberrant retroesophageal right subclavian artery in the adult. *J Thorac Cardiovasc Surg* 61:154–159, 1971.

41. van Son JAM, Vincent JG, ten Cate LN, et al: Anatomic support of surgical approach of anomalous right subclavian artery through a right thoracotomy. *J Thorac Cardiovasc Surg* 99:1115–1116, 1990.

42. Glaevecke, Doehle: Ueber eine seltene angeborene Anomalie der Pulmonalarterie. *Munch Med Wochenschr* 44:950, 1897.

43. Berdon WE, Baker DH, Wung JT, et al: Complete cartilage-ring tracheal stenosis associated with anomalous left pulmonary artery: The ring-sling complex. *Radiology* 152:57–64, 1984.

44. Campbell CD, Wernly JA, Koltip PC, et al: Aberrant left pulmonary artery (pulmonary artery sling): Successful repair and 24 year follow-up report. *Am J Cardiol* 45:316–320, 1980.

45. Grover FL, Norton JB Jr, Webb GE, et al: Pulmonary sling: Case report and collective review. *J Thorac Cardiovasc Surg* 69:295–300, 1975.

46. Koopot R, Nikaidoh H, Idriss FS: Surgical management of anomalous left pulmonary artery causing tracheobronchial obstruction: Pulmonary artery sling. *J Thorac Cardiovasc Surg* 69:239–246, 1975.

47. Backer CL, Idriss FS, Holinger LD, et al: Pulmonary artery sling: Results of surgical repair in infancy. *J Thorac Cardiovasc Surg* 103:683–691, 1992.

48. Jonas RA, Spevak PJ, McGill T, et al: Pulmonary artery sling: Primary

repair by tracheal resection in infancy. *J Thorac Cardiovasc Surg* 97:548–550, 1989.

49. Pawade A, de Leval MR, Elliott MJ, et al: Pulmonary artery sling. *Ann Thorac Surg* 54:967–970, 1992.

50. Benjamin B, Pitkin J, Cohen D: Congenital tracheal stenosis. *Ann Otol Rhinol Laryngol* 90:364–371, 1981.

51. Janik JS, Nagaraj HS, Yacoub U, et al: Congenital funnel-shaped tracheal stenosis: An asymptomatic lethal anomaly of early infancy. *J Thorac Cardiovasc Surg* 83:761–766, 1982.

52. Cantrell JR, Guild HG: Congenital stenosis of the trachea. *Am J Surg* 108:297–305, 1964.

53. Heimansohn DA, Kesler KA, Turrentine MW, et al: Anterior pericardial tracheoplasty for congenital tracheal stenosis. *J Thorac Cardiovasc Surg* 102:710–715, 1991.

54. Nakayama DK, Harrison MR, de Lorimier AA, et al: Reconstructive surgery for obstructing lesions of the intrathoracic trachea in infants and small children. *J Pediatr Surg* 17:854–868, 1982.

55. Jaquiss RDB, Lusk RP, Spray TL, et al: Repair of long-segment tracheal stenosis in infancy. *J Thorac Cardiovasc Surg* 110:1504–1511, 1995.

56. Tsang V, Murday A, Gillbe C, et al: Slide tracheoplasty for congenital funnel-shaped tracheal stenosis. *Ann Thorac Surg* 48:632–635, 1989.

57. Grillo HC: Slide tracheoplasty for long-segment congenital tracheal stenosis. *Ann Thorac Surg* 58:613–619, 1994.

58. Cosentino CM, Backer CL, Idriss FS, et al: Pericardial patch tracheoplasty for severe tracheal stenosis in children: Intermediate results. *J Pediatr Surg* 26:879–884, 1991.

59. Dunham ME, Holinger LD, Backer CL, et al: Management of severe congenital tracheal stenosis. *Ann Otol Rhinol Laryngol* 103:351–356, 1994.

60. Dayan SH, Dunham ME, Backer CL, et al: Slide tracheoplasty in the management of congenital tracheal stenosis. *Ann Otol Rhinol Laryngol,* in press.

61. Backer CL, Mavroudis C, Dunham ME, et al: Repair of congenital tracheal stenosis with a free tracheal autograft, submitted for publication.

62. Backer CL, Mavroudis C, Dunham ME, et al: Reoperation after pericardial patch tracheoplasty. *J Pediatr Surg,* in press.

63. Filler RM, Forte V, Fraga JC, et al: The use of expandable metallic airway stents for tracheobronchial obstruction in children. *J Pediatr Surg* 30:1050–1056, 1995.

64. Burke RP, Chang AC: Video-assisted thoracoscopic division of a vascular ring in an infant: A new operative technique. *J Card Surg* 8:537–540, 1993.

65. Laborde F, Noirhomme P, Karam J, et al: A new video-assisted thoracoscopic surgical technique for interruption of patent ductus arteriosus in infants and children. *J Thorac Cardiovasc Surg* 105:278–280, 1993.

66. Burke RP, Wernovsky G, van der Velde M, et al: Video-assisted thora-

coscopic surgery for congenital heart disease. *J Thorac Cardiovasc Surg* 109:499–508, 1995.

67. Murthy K, Mattioli L, Diehl AM, et al: Vascular ring due to left aortic arch, right descending aorta, and right patent ductus arteriosus. *J Pediatr Surg* 5:550–554, 1970.

68. Whitman G, Stephenson LW, Weinberg P: Vascular ring: Left cervical aortic arch, right descending aorta, and right ligamentum arteriosum. *J Thorac Cardiovasc Surg* 83:311–315, 1982.

69. Park SC, Siewers RD, Neches WH, et al: Left aortic arch with right descending aorta and right ligamentum arteriosum: A rare form of vascular ring. *J Thorac Cardiovasc Surg* 71:779–784, 1976.

70. Watanabe M, Kawasaki S, Sato H, et al: Left aortic arch with right descending aorta and right ligamentum arteriosum associated with d-TGA and large VSD: Surgical treatment of a rare form of vascular ring. *J Pediatr Surg* 30:1363–1365, 1995.

71. McFaul R, Millard P, Nowicki E: Vascular rings necessitating right thoracotomy. *J Thorac Cardiovasc Surg* 82:306–309, 1981.

72. van Son JAM, Julsrud PR, Hagler DJ, et al: Imaging strategies for vascular rings. *Ann Thorac Surg* 57:604–610, 1994.

73. Binet JP, Conso JF, Losay J, et al: Ductus arteriosus sling: Report of a newly recognised anomaly and its surgical correction. *Thorax* 33:72–75, 1978.

74. Ben-Shachar G, Beder SD, Liebman J, et al: Hemitruncal sling: A newly recognized anomaly and its surgical correction. *J Thorac Cardiovasc Surg* 90:146–148, 1985.

CHAPTER 4

Double-Switch Operation for Congenitally Corrected Transposition

Yasuharu Imai, M.D.
Professor and Chairman, Department of Pediatric Cardiovascular
Surgery, The Heart Institute of Japan, Tokyo Women's Medical College,
Tokyo, Japan

Congenitally corrected transposition of the great arteries (CTGA) can be subdivided into 2 groups: congenitally physiologically corrected transposition with atrioventricular discordance, and a much rarer form of anatomically corrected transposition associated with a normal atrioventricular (AV) relationship and with discordant ventriculoarterial (VA) connection. In this chapter, only physiologically corrected transposition is described as CTGA.

Congenitally corrected transposition of the great arteries has unique features in the AV as well as VA arrangements, in which the anatomical right ventricle serves as a systemic ventricle and the anatomical left ventricle functions as a pulmonic counterpart. Although conventional repair yielded excellent results on a short-term basis, long-term systemic right ventricular function remains to be a matter of concern.[1-6] Deterioration of systemic right ventricular function associated with tricuspid regurgitation in cases with complete transposition of the great arteries after Mustard or Senning procedures[7-14] also suggests late deterioration of systemic ventricular function in CTGA with AV discordance. Late postoperative studies in isolated CGTA also revealed systemic right ventricular dysfunction and failure to increase the right ventricular ejection fraction with exercise.[1-3, 7]

Double-switch operation for CTGA has the advantage of creating nearly normal AV and VA relationships, in which the anatomical left ventricle serves as a systemic ventricle and the anatomical right ventricle functions as a pulmonic ventricle postoperatively. The purpose of this chapter is to present the author's series of anatomical repair in CTGA and to compare the postoperative ventricular function of anatomic repair of CTGA with that of the conventional external conduit repair in AV discordance and in complete transposition of the great arteries.

MATERIALS AND METHODS

PATIENT PROFILES

From June, 1989, to August, 1996, 44 patients with CTGA who were younger than 16 years underwent double-switch operations consisting of 31 Mustard or 13 Senning procedures at the atrial level, and 9 arterial switch operations, 22 external conduit repairs, and direct anastomosis between the pulmonary artery and right ventricle in 12 cases at the VA level. In the remaining patient, intraventricular rerouting along with the Senning procedure was performed to complete anatomical correction (Table 1). The Mustard procedure with patch augmentation of the functional systemic atrium was selected for a small right atrium, and arterial switch in cases with intact pulmonary valves (Table 2).

There were 30 males and 14 females. Ages at operation ranged from 3 months to 15 years (mean, 7.1 ± 3.5 years), and body weights ranged from 4.6 to 49 kg (mean, 20.1 ± 9.0 kg). Before the double-switch operation, palliative procedures were performed 54 times in 33 patients; these consisted of systemic-to-pulmonary shunts and pulmonary banding including 42 shunt procedures, and 8 pulmonary artery banding procedures for preparation of anatomical left ventricle in 3 cases, or for control of pulmonary hypertension in 4 cases (Table 3). A 2-year-old boy who had grade-3 sys-

---

TABLE 1.
Double-Switch Procedures

Atrial Switch	No. of Cases	Ventriculoarterial Switch	No. of Cases
Mustard	31	External conduit repair	22
		Direct PA-RV anastomosis	12
Senning	13	Arterial switch	9
		Intraventricular conduit	1

Abbreviations: PA, pulmonary artery; RV, right ventricle.

TABLE 2.
Direction of Cardiac Apex and Atrial Switch
Procedure

Atrial Switch	Normal Direction	Meso-Position	Opposite Direction
Senning (13 cases)	10	2	1
Mustard (31 cases)	1	6	24

TABLE 3.
Previous Palliation (54 Times in 33 Patients)

Palliative Procedures (33 cases)	No. of Procedures
Blalock-Taussig shunt	
Modified	21
Original	16
Central shunt	2
with angioplasty	2
Waterston shunt	1
Pulmonary banding	
for LV training	4
for PH	3
with coarctation repair	1
Unifocalization of MAPCA	2
Miscellaneous	2

Abbreviations: LV, left ventricular; *PH,* pulmonary hypertension; *MAPCA,* major aortopulmonary collateral artery.

temic tricuspid regurgitation associated with a small ventricular septal defect (VSD), underwent two successive pulmonary arterial banding procedures for preparation of the left ventricle 7 months before the anatomical correction. Pulmonary artery banding resulted in spontaneous closure of the VSD and reduction in tricuspid regurgitation at the time of double-switch operation.

Associated anomalies were seen in all cases, consisting of VSD in 41 cases, atrial septal defect in 16, pulmonary atresia in 21, pulmonary stenosis in 14, bilateral superior vena cava in 9, patent duc-

TABLE 4.
Associated Anomalies and Complications

Anomalies and Complications	No. Cases	Anomalies and Complications	No. Cases
VSD	41	Systemic TR	20
ASD	16	MR	12
PFO	13	Ebstein's anomaly	1
PDA	6	WPW	2
Pulmonary atresia	21	PSVT	3
Pulmonary stenosis	14	Complete AV block	1
Pulmonary hypertension	4	Single coronary artery	4
PA coarctation	12	MAPCA	1
Nonconfluent PA	2	Aortic coarctation with SAS	1
Bilateral SVC	9	AR	3
Absent ipsilateral SVC	1	PAPVC	1

Abbreviations: VSD, ventricular septal defect; *ASD,* atrial septal defect, *PFO,* patent foramen ovale; *PDA,* patent ductus arteriosus; *PA,* pulmonary artery; *SVC,* superior vena cava; *TR,* tricuspid regurgitation; *WPW,* Wolff-Parkinson-White syndrome; *PSVT,* paroxysmal supraventricular tachycardia; *AV,* atrioventricular; *MAPCA;* major aortopulmonary collateral artery; *SAS,* subaortic stenosis; *AR,* aortic regurgitation; *PAPVC,* partial anomalous pulmonary venous connection.

tus arteriosus in 6, Wolff-Parkinson-White syndrome (WPW) in 2, congenital AV block in 1, and single coronary artery in 4. Systemic tricuspid regurgitation (TR) was seen in 20 patients, mitral regurgitation (MR) in 12, and aortic regurgitation (AR) in 4 patients (Table 4). Situs solitus (SDD) was seen in 29 and inverted situs (ILL) in 15 patients.

Risk factors regarding application of conventional repair by using the systemic right ventricle were observed in 28 of 44 patients (64%), including systemic TR in 20 cases, poor right ventricular ejection fraction in 10, small right ventricular volume in 3, or large right ventricular volume in 6 (Table 5).

CATHETERIZATION STUDIES
Left and right ventricular function were evaluated by cineangiogram before and approximately 1–3 months after operation (range, 18 days to 18 months [98.7 ± 148.9 days]). The volume of the morphologic left ventricle (LV) was calculated with the area-length method, and that of the morphologic right ventricle (RV)

TABLE 5.
Risk Factors for Conventional Repair (30 Cases With Risk Factors)

Case No.	TR grade (Seller)	RVEDV <80% of normal	RVEDV >200%	RVEF <50%	RVEDP ≤14 mm Hg
1	3		213		
2	3			41	14
3		74			
5	2				
6	2				
7	1		241		
8	1	74			
9	1				
10				42	
11		62			
12	1				
15				42	
16	1				
20			206		
21	4		244	39	21
22	2		230		
25	4		254	41	
26				46	
33	1				
36	1			48	17
37	3				
38	2			43	
39				45	
40	2				
41				41	
42	1				
43	1				
44	1				
TOTAL	20	3	6	10	3

Abbreviations: TR, tricuspid regurgitation; *RVEDV*, right ventricular end-diastolic volume; *RVEF*, right ventricular ejection fraction; *RVEDP*, right ventricular end-diastolic pressure.

with Simpson's rule by the method of Graham et al.[15] Adjustment
of volume occupied by papillary muscles for the left ventricle was
made according to Graham et al.[16] as follows: When the measured
volume of LV (V) was less than 15 mL, adjusted LV volume (V') =
0.874V−3.1 was applied, and for LV volume more than 15 mL,
V' = 0.733V was applied. Similarly, for the morphologic RV calculated by Simpson's method, adjustment was made by the following formula: V' = 0.649V. Both adjusted ventricular volumes were
then expressed as a percentage of the expected normal ventricular
volume of each respective ventricle per body surface area (BSA)
according to the formula by Nakazawa et al. as follows[17]:

Normal left ventricular end-diastolic volume (LVEDV)
$$= 72.5 \times BSA1.43$$
Normal right ventricular end-diastolic volume (RVEDV)
$$= 75.1 \times BSA1.43$$

Postoperatively, pulmonic ventricular volume and its ejection
fraction were calculated by excluding the subvalvular portion of
external conduits in all types of external conduit repair both in conventional repair and in double-switch operation. Regarding stroke
volume index, commonly expressed as milliliters per square meter
of BSA, ventricular end-diastolic volume (expressed as a percentage of normal value) multiplied by ejection fraction is arbitrarily
termed as % stroke volume index in this chapter for the sake of
standardization and ease of comparison. All mean values are expressed as a mean ± 1 SD, and a paired or unpaired t test was used
for statistical analysis.

The preoperative ratio of left and right systolic ventricular pressures ranged from 0.78 to 1.17 (mean, 1.0 ± 0.07), the cardiothoracic ratio averaged 50.3 ± 5.9% (range, 38% to 63%), the PA
index[18] ranged from 126 to 930mm^2/m^2 (mean, 346.1 ± 146.4
mm^2/m^2), the systemic arterial partial pressure of oxygen (Pao$_2$)
ranged from 27 to 88 mm Hg (mean, 45.2 ± 15.5 mm Hg), the systemic arterial oxygen saturation ranged from 48% to 97% (mean,
78.3 ± 11.2%), and the pulmonary-to-systemic flow ratio (Qp/Qs)
ranged from 0.33 to 4.6 (mean, 1.1 ± 0.7). The preoperative systemic RVEDV ranged from 62% to 244% (mean, 129.5 ± 44.1%),
the right ventricular ejection fraction (RVEF) ranged from 39% to
77% (mean, 55 ± 8%), the pulmonic LVEDV ranged from 75% to
269% (mean, 134.0 ± 48.1%), and the left ventricular ejection fraction (LVEF) ranged from 40% to 75% (mean, 61 ± 7%).

Postoperative catheterization and angiography was performed

in 31 patients ranging from 18 days to 18 months (mean, 98.7 ±
148.9 days) after operation.

The systemic ventricular function after double-switch operation was compared with that of conventional external conduit repair bridging between the left ventricular apex and the pulmonary
artery in 20 cases with CTGA in our series. Also, ventricular function after double-switch operation, consisting of external conduit
repair combined with Mustard or Senning procedure, was compared with ventricular function in 23 cases of complete transposition (TGA) with VSD and with reduced pulmonary blood flow in
which external conduit repair was performed in our institution
during approximately the same period.

SURGICAL TECHNIQUES

Intracardiac repair was performed through a median sternotomy
using moderately hypothermic cardiopulmonary bypass (25° C to
27° C) via ascending aortic and direct bicaval or tricaval cannulation. Glucose-insulin-potassium solution (20 mL/kg) was used to
induce cardioplegia and was administered in half the dose every
40 minutes thereafter. For the atrial switch procedure, the Senning
repair was preferred in cases with a normal or large right atrium.
The Mustard procedure with liberal patch augmentation of the
functional left atrium, on the other hand, was chosen for cases in
which there was a small right atrium resulting from an overhang-
ing anatomical left ventricle in mesocardia or dextrocardia in situs
solitus. At the VA level, the arterial switch operation was performed in cases with normal pulmonary valves, and external conduit repair with intraventricular rerouting was preferred for pulmonary atresia or pulmonary valvular stenosis in our earlier series.
However, in our recent series, right ventricular outflow reconstruction with a monocusp patch was performed after direct anastomosis between the RV and distal pulmonary artery in an attempt to
eliminate the external conduit. In case 39, CTGA associated with
superoinferior ventricular relationship, DORV in SLD (situs solitus, L-loop, d-transposition) and single left coronary artery following pulmonary artery banding, intraventricular conduit repair was
feasible by making an intraventricular route between a large VSD
and aorta to complete the anatomical repair.

Thus, the combinations of double-switch procedures were as
follows: Mustard and external conduit repair in 18 cases, Mustard
and direct anastomosis in 10, Senning and external conduit repair
in 4, Senning and direct anastomosis in 2, Mustard and arterial

switch operation in 3, Senning with arterial switch in 6, and Senning with intraventricular conduit in 1 case (Table 6).

ATRIAL SWITCH PROCEDURES

The Mustard procedure was performed through a vertical incision in the right atrium, and an additional transverse incision was made toward the confluence of right pulmonary veins to create a T-shaped opening. After liberal atrial septectomy, a systemic venous channel was created with a glutaraldehyde-treated equine pericardial baffle (Xenomedica). The ostium of the coronary sinus was always incorporated in the systemic venous channel, because an anterior conduction system was the rule in CTGA, unless proven otherwise. In cases with bilateral superior vena cava (SVC), the coronary sinus was cut back deep into the left atrium, and its cranial wall was used as a pedicled flap to partially create a ceiling of the pulmonary venous channel in 7 patients (cases 2, 9, 11, 25, 33, 34, and 43). Similarly in case 3, partial pulmonary venous return into the right SVC was corrected by diverting the inferior vena cava, and persistent left SVC into anatomical left atrium by a partial Mustard baffle, in which the ostium of right SVC into the anatomical right atrium was kept and the right SVC distal to the anomalous pulmonary venous connection was ligated. In all Mustard cases, the functional left atrium was deliberately enlarged with Xenomedica membrane or autologous pericardial patch down to the confluence of right pulmonary veins.

In Senning cases, the standard Senning procedure was performed in 11 patients (cases 1, 4, 8, 12, 22, 26, 37, 38, 39, 42, and

TABLE 6.
Combination of Double-Switch Procedures and Results

Ventriculo arterial level	Mustard No. Cases	Senning No. Cases	Total
External conduit repair	18 (2)*	4	22 (2)
Direct PA-RV anastomosis	10 (1)	2	12 (1)
Arterial switch operation	3 (1)	6	9 (1)
Intraventricular conduit repair		1	1
Total	31 (4)	13	44 (4)

*Number of deaths in parentheses.
Abbreviations: PA, pulmonary artery; *RV*, right ventricular.

44), and cut-back of the coronary sinus in cases with the persistent contralateral SVC was added in cases 5 and 7.

SWITCH PROCEDURES AT VENTRICULOARTERIAL LEVEL

Arterial Switch Operation

The arterial switch operation using the French maneuver in the presence of a normal pulmonary valve was performed in cases 1, 2, 7, 21, 22, 25, 37, 38, and 44. Closure of the VSD was generally performed through the right atrial approach or through combined right atrial and transaortic routes in one patient. Pledgeted-mattress sutures were used exclusively in all cases. Those sutures were placed on the anatomical right ventricular side along the cranial and anterior margin of the defect, and on the margin of the left ventricular aspect of the ventricular septum on its posterior margin, when closure of the VSD was performed through the right atrial approach. Mirror-images of the normal coronary pattern were seen in all cases, and round coronary buttons were translocated into punched-out holes in the facing wall of the pulmonary artery above the level of the sinus Valsalva. Coronary defects in the old aortic root were closed with two autologous pericardial patches.

External Conduit Repair

In external conduit repair, ventricular rerouting was performed with a double-layer Xenomedica membrane, or with a composite patch of thin Dacron velour and Xenomedica membrane. Fixation of intraventricular conduit was also done using pledgeted-mattress sutures placed exclusively on the right ventricular side of the ventricular septum and then onto the aortic valve ring mainly using a running suture. Along the posterior margin of the defect, sutures were placed through the tricuspid valve ring and then directly on the margin of the VSD, disregarding the possibility of the posterior conduction system regardless of the visceral situs and of the VA connection, unless evidence existed for posterior conduction, proved by electrophysiologic study (EPS) before operation. Complete AV block occurred in one case of situs inversus (IDD) (case 31), in which enlargement of the VSD was done by resecting its posterior margin. Therefore, preoperative EPS seemed advisable especially in CTGA in the inverted situs. There were 15 cases with CTGA in situs inversus (IDD type) in this series, and 13 of them underwent closure of VSD or intraventricular rerouting disregarding the possibility of posterior conduction. In the remaining patient, posterior conduction was verified by preoperative EPS. Thus, presence of the posterior conduction system was proved only in 2 of 15 cases (13%) despite conventional knowledge that the posterior conduction was a rule in CTGA in situs inversus.

Ventricular Septal Defect

A VSD extending from the membranous septum to the aortic valve ring without a recognizable infundibular septum (total conus defect in our classification) was the best indication for rerouting, and this favorable type of VSD was seen in 4 of 35 cases undergoing intraventricular rerouting (cases 3, 9, 16, and 41). Two other patients had a VSD without a distal infundibular septum and with a muscular margin proximally (distal conus defect). In the remaining 29 cases, a VSD was located in the membranous portion of the septum with various degrees of infundibular extension—as seen in patients with the ordinary tetralogy of Fallot (25 cases) and the remaining 4 cases (cases 13 18, 19, and 20), in which the defect was located in the middle of the infundibular septum (midconus defect according to our classification, or infundibular muscular defect). Provided the anterior conduction system was present in all cases, carving of its protrusion on the RV side could be done safely. The outlet portion of the septum was generally composed of infundibular septum and the original ventricular septum, in which the former covered the cranial aspect of the VSD on the RV side. Because the infundibular septum should not contain a conduction system, its resection could be done safely. It was our practice to look at the anatomical composition of the VSD in the LV aspect through an RA approach. Along the anterior margin of the VSD, the lower margin of the infundibular septum could be recognized not infrequently as a second margin on the opposite side of the septum restricting VSD. This portion of the infundibular septum could be resected. Also, wedge resection of the ventricular septum proper at the posterocaudal corner of the VSD was naturally possible. In cases with double-outlet right ventricle with CTGA with or without pulmonary atresia, resection of the infundibular septum also could be performed after analyzing the structure on the LV surface. Enlargement of the VSD, including carving of the infundibular septum, was necessary in 15 patients, and in only 1 patient (case 31) did surgical AV block develop.

Right Ventricle Outflow Reconstruction by Direct Anastomosis

Extracardiac conduit bearing 3 cusps was handmade on the table using Xenomedica membrane in 15 cases.[19] In the recent 7 cases, the conduit made of the autologous pericardium bearing a monocusp was used instead. Diameters of the conduit ranged from 20 to

26 mm. Because the Xenomedica conduit had limited durability and required reoperation for conduit stenosis in 5–10 years in our series of the conduit repair in the other complex anomalies, right ventricular reconstruction by direct anastomosis between the pulmonary artery and right ventricular incision was performed whenever possible in the recent series. In 12 patients, the distal end of the pulmonary artery was brought down to the cranial margin of the right ventriculotomy to the left of the aorta in situs solitus and to the right in situs inversus. Then direct anastomosis was performed to create an autologous posterior wall of the outflow tract, which was then enlarged with an autologous pericardial patch bearing a monocusp. This type of direct anastomosis was feasible almost always in cases with relatively well-developed confluent pulmonary artery by mobilizing both pulmonary branches beyond the hilar level, similar to the arterial switch operation. To approximate a gap between the distal pulmonary stump and RV incision, an appropriate pedicled flap was developed in the pulmonary artery by making an oblique incision in its anterior wall extending into the left pulmonary artery, and the left proximal corner of the incision was flipped over to reach the cranial end of the RV incision. The direct anastomosis was performed with a running 6-0 or 5-0 absorbable suture reinforced with one or two additional pledgeted-mattress sutures if required.

REPAIR OF ATRIOVENTRICULAR VALVE AND OTHER CONCOMITANT PROCEDURES

Mitral regurgitation resulting from a cleft anterior leaflet was repaired by suture closure and annuloplasty in cases 2, 3, and 4. Mitral valve replacement with a 23-mm St. Jude Medical valve had to be done in case 2 after unsuccessful valve repair.

Mild-to-severe systemic tricuspid regurgitation was seen in 20 patients preoperatively, and Reed's tricuspid annuloplasty was performed in 5 cases at the commissure between septal and posterior leaflets.

The accessory pathway was confirmed between the left atrium and anatomical RV by epicardial mapping, and Sealy's operation combined with cryoablation for type A WPW syndrome was performed in cases 5 and 6. In case 15, repeated episodes of paroxysmal supraventricular tachycardia were controlled by Sealy's operation and cryoablation, and prosthetic aortic valve replacement with a 19-mm St. Jude Medical valve was also performed. In case 1, pacemaker implantation was done for congenital AV block.

TABLE 7.
Perfusion Time and Aortic Cross Clamp Time in 44
Patients

	Mean* (Minute)	Range (Minute)
Perfusion time	239.5 ± 37.4	176–339
Aortic clamp time†	92.2 ± 35.1	45–189

*Mean: mean ± 1 standard deviation.
†Aortic clamp time: aortic cross clamp time.

RESULTS

These procedures are complex. The aortic cross clamp times and cardiopulmonary bypass times are noted in Table 7.

All but four patients survived the operation, and the hospital mortality rate was 9.1%. The patient in case 2 died of low cardiac output caused by massive regurgitation of the neoaortic valve; in case 17, of pulmonary hypertension and septicemia; in case 33, of low cardiac output with acute renal failure; and in case 44, of chronic respiratory failure and pneumonitis caused by tracheo-esophageal fistula of unknown etiology on days 3, 33, 5, and 94 after the operation, respectively. In case 17 associated with pulmonary atresia, preoperative measurement of pulmonary vascular resistance index (PVRI) was erroneous. Pulmonary mean arterial pressure measured by insertion of a catheter through a Blalock-Taussig shunt yielded a low pressure of 8 mm Hg, and the resultant PVRI was reported to be 1.3 Wood's units. However, postoperative catheterization disclosed prohibitive PVRI of 9.3 Wood's units. Preoperative catheterization data were re-evaluated. Left pulmonary venous wedge pressure was found elevated (33 mm Hg), and PVRI was corrected to be 9.4 Wood's units, with which total correction should have been contraindicated.

Follow-up in 40 survivors ranged from 1 to 87 months (mean, 3.0 ± 2.2 years). At the time that this manuscript was written, 35 patients were in New York Heart Association (NYHA) functional class 1, 3 patients were in class 2, and 2 were still in the recuperating period after the operation in our hospital. Reoperation for repair of superior vena caval obstruction 1 month after operation was performed in case 10, and closure of residual shunts both at the atrial and ventricular level 31 months later was performed in case 4. Two had permanent surgical AV block after double-switch operation (cases 31 and 44). Regarding residual regurgitation of AV valves, postoperative tricuspid regurgitation was grade 1/4 in 8 patients and 2/4 in 1 patient by cineangiogram. Systemic mitral regurgitation was grade 1/4 in 10 cases and 2/4 in 1 patient on cineangiogram.

POSTOPERATIVE PARAMETERS

After double-switch operation, the cardiothoracic ratio increased from 50.3 ± 5.9% to 57.7 ± 5.5% postoperatively ($P = 0.0001$). Anatomical RVEDV showed a significant reduction from 129.5 ± 44.1% of normal to 95.0 ± 37.1%, resulting from unloading of the ventricle and diversion of its outflow tract into the systemic ventricular outlet by intraventricular rerouting after operation ($P = 0.0002$), and the RVEF remained unchanged (55 ± 8% to 54 ± 6%). Postoperatively systolic pressure in the RV showed a marked decrease to 44.7 ± 15.2 mm Hg, and RV-to-LV systolic pressure ratio decreased to 0.46 ± 0.17. Anatomical LVEDV remained unchanged before and after operation; 134.0 ± 48.1% of normal vs. 135.2 ± 45.3% ($P = 0.7756$), respectively. The LVEF showed a significant decrease from 61 ± 7% to 54 ± 10% ($P = 0.002$); however, it remained within the normal range in the majority of the cases. The cardiac index averaged 3.1 ± 0.6 L/m^2 after surgery (range 2.0–4.4 L/m^2). Changes in LVEF before and after double-switch operation showed an increase in 10 cases, a decrease in 19 patients, and remained the same in one patient (Fig 1). In 6 patients (cases 4, 6, 11, 12, 16, and 18), medium-term follow-up catheterization 1–1.5 years after operation was performed. In case 6, LVEF increased from 0.42 at 1 month after surgery to 0.50 at 1 year, and the cardiac index also showed an increase from 2.6 to 3.4 L/min/m^2. In the other 2 cases, exercise testing by supine bicycle ergometer was performed during catheterization. Marked increases in cardiac output compared with the resting state were observed. Cardiac indices increased from 3.3 and 3.0 L/min/m^2 at rest to 5.5 and 4.6 L/min/m^2 after exercise in cases 11 and 12, respectively.

Comparison With Conventional Repair in Congenitally Corrected Transposition of the Great Arteries

Systemic ventricular function after double-switch operation was compared with that of conventional external conduit repair between LV apex and pulmonary artery in 20 patients younger than 16 years with CTGA. Although systemic ventricular end-diastolic pressure (11.9 ± 5.5 vs. 12.9 ± 3.5 mm Hg), systemic ventricular end-diastolic volume (127.3 ± 32.8% vs. 104.5 ± 24.9%), systemic

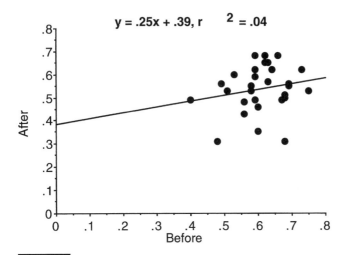

FIGURE 1.
Left ventricular ejection fraction (LVEF) before and after double-switch operation. The LVEF showed an insignificant decrease after operation but remained within normal limits in the majority of cases. *Abbreviation: NS, not significant.*

ventricular ejection fraction (0.56 ± 10% vs. 0.53 ± 0.06%), and systemic % stroke volume index (66.5 ± 13.3% vs. 55.5 ± 15.0%) were statistically insignificant, all parameters of systemic ventricular function suggested better performance after the double-switch operation.

Comparison With Transposition of the Great Arteries

When ventricular function after double-switch operation consisting of external conduit repair combined with Mustard or Senning procedure was compared with that in 23 cases of complete transposition of the great arteries (TGA) with VSD and with reduced pulmonary blood flow after external conduit repair, right atrial pressure (10.0 ± 5.5 mm Hg vs. 8.4 ± 3.7 mm Hg), LV end-diastolic pressure (12.9 ± 4.8 mm Hg vs. 10.6 ± 4.0 mm Hg), pressure gradient between LV and aorta (2.5 ± 5.3 mm Hg vs. 3.3 ± 4.2 mm Hg), pressure gradient between RV and distal PA (13.6 ± 13.5 mm Hg vs. 16.9 ± 11.3 mm Hg), RV/LV peak systolic pressure ratio (0.48 ± 0.21 vs. 0.51 ± 0.14), RVEF (0.57 ± 0.06 vs. 0.55 ± 0.09), and LVEF (0.56 ± 0.1 vs. 0.56 ± 0.09) were statistically insignificant. However, cardiac index (3.2 ± 0.5 L/m^2 vs. 3.7 ± 0.8 L/m^2, P = 0.0359), RVEDV (72.7 ± 19.4% vs. 115.7 ± 47.0%, P = 0.0048), RV % stroke volume index (41.1 ± 11.2% vs. 62.3 ± 23.3%, $P = 0.0056$), LVEDV (122.5 ± 28.5% vs. 170.5 ± 45.1%, $P = 0.0015$), and LV % stroke volume index (66.5 ± 13.3% vs. 94.1 ± 22.5%, $P = 0.0003$) were significantly larger in the TGA group. These significant differences in ventricular volume in the two groups were merely a reflection of increased volumes before operation in the TGA group. Preoperatively, RVEDV, RV % stroke volume index, LVEDV, and LV % stroke volume index in the TGA group were already larger than those in the CTGA group: RVEDV (140.5 ± 41.7% vs. 106.7 ± 26.6%, $P = 0.0084$), RV % stroke volume index (80.0 ± 21.2% vs. 60.1 ± 15.2%, $P = 0.0034$), LVEDV (164.3 ± 62.3% vs. 119.9 ± 35.2%, $P = 0.0169$), and LV % stroke volume index (99.6 ± 36.6% vs. 73.2 ± 25.5%, $P = 0.0205$). These significant differences in ventricular volumes in the two groups before operation resulted from younger age at operation and to higher Qp/Qs in the TGA group.

Postoperative increases in LV volume after Rastelli-type repair were observed both in the TGA and double-switch groups. Ratios of LVEDV before and after operation were 113 ± 26% of preoperative value in the TGA and 108 ± 28% in the double-switch group. These increases in LVEDV were accompanied by a corresponding reduction in RVEDV after operation. Ratios of RVEDV before and after surgery were 86 ± 28% in the TGA and 67 ± 18% in the double-switch group. Because the volume occupied by the intraventricular conduit, which was located in the outflow portion of the anatomical RV, was inevitably added to the postoperative LVEDV and the same amount had to be subtracted from RVEDV, at least part of the changes in ventricular volumes would be caused by this mechanism besides the unloading effect on RVEDV and diminution in tricuspid regurgitation.

Arterial Switch Operation

In five of eight surviving patients after combined atrial switch and arterial switch operation, postoperative catheterization was performed. The RVEDV showed a marked decrease from 191.1 ± 41.9% to 118 ± 37.3% of normal ($P = 0.003$) resulting from the unloading effect after operation. Postoperative systemic LV function revealed satisfactory results. Although LVEDV remained unchanged (183.7 ± 64.9% of normal before operation to 192.8 ± 60.8% of normal after operation, $P = 0.7104$), and LVEF decreased insignificantly (from 61 ± 8% to 49 ± 1%, $P = 0.0534$), the cardiac index was 3.1 ± 0.5 L/min/m^2 (range, 2.3–3.6 L/min/m^2), and all but one patient were in NYHA class 1 at the time of this writing. Postoperative LVEF in this subset remained greater than 50% in four of five patients studied; only one case after LV training by PA banding showed a rather drastic reduction in LVEF after operation—from 48% to 31%.

DISCUSSION

BACKGROUND

The long-term outcome of the anatomical right ventricle as a systemic ventricle still remains controversial in patients with CTGA associated with AV discordance.[1-6] Systemic right ventricular failure usually associated with tricuspid regurgitation after Mustard or Senning procedures in complete transposition of the great arteries is seen with increasing frequency,[7-14] and the failing right ventricular function can be normalized by conversion from atrial switch to arterial switch operation. Also, the author's clinical experience in conversion of atrial switch to arterial switch after systemic RV failure in TGA in six cases, in which five patients survived and were doing well, showed that the systemic LV greatly improved the quality of life of these patients. Because systemic right ventricular function rapidly deteriorates in association with tricuspid regurgitation, and the tricuspid regurgitation of systemic right ventricle presents as one of the major risk factors in conventional surgical correction of associated anomalies in CTGA,[1,6] the double-switch operation or anatomical correction carries the best hope in terms of patients' longevity.

Anatomical correction in CTGA as a combined atrial switch and Rastelli repair has been reported by Ilbawi et al.[20] in 1990 and by Di Donato et al.[21] in 1992. Combined arterial switch and atrial repair as an anatomical repair for AV discordance has never been reported before our study.[22] In the author's series, the first case of double-switch operation consisting of Senning and arterial switch operation was successfully performed on a 2-year-old boy with CTGA associated with grade-3 tricuspid regurgitation on June 12, 1989, and combined Mustard- and Rastelli-type repair was then successfully performed on May 25, 1990. In 1992, direct anastomosis between the distal pulmonary artery and cranial margin of right ventriculotomy was also successfully performed, and this modification similar to réparation à l'étage ventriculairé (REV) in TGA reported by Lecompte would further reduce long-term morbidity and need for reoperation by eliminating a tubular prosthetic material in the outflow reconstruction.[23] Two types of anatomical repair, combined arterial switch and Senning procedure, and combined atrial switch and direct anastomosis between RV and the distal pulmonary artery, seemed to be new combinations (i.e., they had never been performed for CTGA).

HEMODYNAMICS

Because hemodynamic parameters and ventricular function after double-switch operation in CTGA are similar to those in the group with TGA complete transposition of the great arteries after conventional Rastelli-type repair in terms of right atrial pressure, LV end-diastolic pressure, pressure gradient between LV and aorta, RV/LV peak systolic pressure ratio, RVEF, and LVEF, further application of anatomical repair in CTGA seems to be justified. The LVEF at 1 month after operation was lower than normal in 5 of 16 cases studied. The author's normal value for LVEF is 0.63 ± 0.05 (mean $\pm$ SD), and normal range (mean $\pm$ 2 SD) is set between 0.53 and 0.73. However, the fact that the medium-term results in three patients showed improved LV function and a favorable increase in cardiac output and LVEF after exercise would indicate that temporary depression of LV function in the immediate postoperative period could improve. In comparison with the conventional Rastelli procedure in TGA, the LVEF in both groups was exactly the same, and the decrease in LVEF after conduit repair was partly the result of a new addition of noncontractile intraventricular conduit to the left ventricular volume. Also, that all the patients are currently leading normal lives in NYHA classes 1 or 2 encourages us to continue the anatomical correction in CTGA.

ARTERIAL SWITCH OPERATION

Combined atrial and arterial switch operation is preferable over conventional repair in patients with tricuspid regurgitation, because conversion of the systemic RV to a pulmonic ventricle even without direct surgical intervention on the tricuspid valve provides an excellent solution to a hitherto complicated problem. In five of eight surviving patients after combined atrial switch and arterial switch operation, postoperative catheterization was performed. The RVEDV showed a marked decrease from $191.1 \pm 41.9\%$ to $118 \pm 37.3\%$ of normal ($P = 0.003$) as a result of the unloading effect after operation. Postoperative systemic LV function revealed satisfactory results. Although LVEDV remained unchanged before and after operation, from ($183.7 \pm 64.9\%$ of normal before operation to $192.8 \pm 60.8\%$ of normal after operation, $P = 0.7104$), and LVEF decreased insignificantly (from $61 \pm 8\%$ to $49 \pm 1\%$, $P = 0.0534$), the cardiac index was 3.1 ± 0.5 L/min/m^2 (range, 2.3–3.6 L/min/m^2), and all but one patient were in NYHA class 1 at the time of this writing.

However, massive neoaortic regurgitation seen in case 2 with subvalvular pulmonary stenosis contraindicates conversion of an untrained low-pressure pulmonic valve into a neoaortic valve. Because the combination of arterial switch and Senning procedure resulted in excellent systemic LV function after operation, universal application of this type of anatomical repair should be considered in cases with CTGA associated with VSD and pulmonary hypertension in the future.

CORONARY PATTERN

The standard coronary pattern in CTGA with AV discordance is a mirror image of normal. All 9 cases of double-switch operation with arterial switch had the mirror-image pattern in this series, and coronary transfer was feasible without difficulty. However, 4 of 44 patients in this series had a single coronary artery, of which 3 were single anatomical left coronary arteries and one had a single anatomical right coronary artery. On the other hand, only 1 of 79 patients with CTGA in our series of conventional total correction excluding double-switch operation showed an anomalous coronary pattern of single anatomical left coronary artery. Therefore, the overall incidence of anomalous coronary arterial pattern was only 4% (5/123), and it showed a sharp contrast to the high incidence of anomalous patterns in those with TGA who underwent arterial switch operation. The incidence of anomalous coronary patterns in TGA was 28% (96/341) in the author's series, when the standard pattern in this subset was considered to be Shaher type 1, in which the right coronary artery originated from the right-hand sinus and the left counterpart from the left-hand sinus of the aorta supplying the left anterior descending and circumflex branches.

TRICUSPID REGURGITATION

Systemic tricuspid regurgitation was considered to be a major risk and problem in surgical treatment of CTGA, and Ebstein's anomaly of the systemic AV valve was not amenable to conventional valvuloplasty.[1,24–26] Also, postoperative tricuspid regurgitation was clinically insignificant in all cases including one with Ebstein-like anomaly despite the simple application of tricuspid annuloplasty in 5 of 20 cases with preoperative tricuspid regurgitation. Significant reductions in both the end-diastolic volume and peak systolic pressure after the double-switch operation made the previously incompetent tricuspid valve competent. Although longer follow-up is warranted, double-switch operation should be considered best for CTGA, especially when systemic tricuspid regurgitation is present or in cases with poor systemic RV function.

VENTRICULAR SEPTAL DEFECT AND THE CONDUCTION SYSTEM

The location and size of the VSD were important in this type of repair. In isolated VSD in CTGA, typical perimembranous VSD with a long infundibular septum had been seen frequently in the author's experience. However, in cyanotic patients with CTGA, some degree of infundibular extension of VSD seemed to be the rule, partly because of deviation of the infundibular septum toward the pulmonary artery in cases with pulmonic stenosis, or because of maldevelopment of the infundibulum in cases with DORV and pulmonary atresia.[27] This infundibular extension of varying degree is not necessarily unique in Asian populations and is also clearly shown on the angiogram reported by Ilbawi and associates.[20] In cyanotic patients, ejection by the anatomical LV into the left anteriorly placed aorta predisposed straight alignment of the ventricle to the aorta, resulting in dextrocardia or mesocardia in its cardiac position in situs solitus, d-loop, and l-transposition (SLL) and in levocardia or mesocardia in situs inversus, d-loop, and d-transposition (IDD) group.

CONDUCTION SYSTEM AND POSTOPERATIVE ARRHYTHMIA

There is general agreement in the anterior conduction system in SLL group[28]; on the other hand, the posterior conduction system has been reported in CTGA in situs inversus.[29,30] In the author's series of CTGA including conventional Rastelli repair, there were 19 cases of IDD type, in which VSD was either closed or included in the intraventricular conduit. The anterior conduction system was merely preserved and the presence of the posterior counterpart was disregarded in all but one patient, whose conduction system had been proved as the posterior conduction preoperatively. However, sinus rhythm could be maintained in 18 cases after operation. Because there was no difference in AV septal alignment either in SLL or in IDD, anatomical explanation seemed lacking to support a different conduction pattern in all cases of IDD. However, there was a possibility of the dual pathway forming a sling in CTGA, and the exact incidence of the posterior conduction in a large series of cases, especially with a good AV septal alignment, should be studied in detail. Regarding patients with WPW syndrome or preoperative paroxysmal supraventricular tachycardia (PSVT), recurrence of tachyarrhythmia was seen in case 7 and was controlled with antiarrhythmic medication. In the remaining two patients, arrhythmia surgery combined with cryoablation successfully abolished recurrence.

SUMMARY

Since June, 1989, 44 patients with congenitally corrected transposition associated with AV discordance who were younger than 16 years underwent anatomical correction, or double-switch operation; 4 of the patients (9.1%) died while still hospitalized. Although double-switch operation is a time-consuming procedure, and longer follow-up is warranted, it is best indicated for CTGA, especially in the presence of systemic tricuspid regurgitation, or in cases with poor systemic RV function. Preoperative tricuspid regurgitation improved spontaneously without surgical intervention on the valve, and mere unloading of the anatomical RV was proven sufficient to control the regurgitation in our series. Postoperative ventricular function can be favorably compared with that of the conventional Rastelli procedure in the complete transposition of the great arteries. Combined atrial switch and arterial switch procedures were performed in nine cases, and eight surviving patients were currently doing well in NYHA functional class 1 at the time this report was written. This combination of anatomical repair should be considered for cases with CTGA associated with VSD and pulmonary hypertension. Two types of anatomical repair that the author first described, combined arterial switch and the Senning procedure, and combined atrial switch and direct anastomosis between the RV and the distal pulmonary artery, seemed to be preferable methods for performing anatomical correction in CTGA.

REFERENCES

1. McGrath LB, Kirklin JW, Blackstone EH, et al: Death and other events after cardiac repair in discordant atrioventricular connection. *J Thorac Cardiovasc Surg* 90:711–728, 1985.
2. Graham TP, Parrish MD, Boncek RJ, et al: Assessment of ventricular size and function in congenitally corrected transposition of the great arteries. *Am J Cardiol* 54:244–251, 1983.
3. Peterson RJ, Franch RH, Fajman WA, et al: Comparison of cardiac function in surgically corrected and congenitally corrected transposition of the great arteries. *J Thorac Cardiovasc Surg* 96:227–236, 1988.
4. Dimas AP, Moodie DS, Sterba R, et al: Long-term function of the morphologic right ventricle in adult patients with corrected transposition of the great arteries. *Am Heart J* 118:526–530, 1989.
5. Benson LN, Burns R, Schwaiger M, et al: Radionuclide angiographic evaluation of ventricular function in isolated congenitally corrected transposition of the great arteries. *Am J Cardiol* 58:319–324, 1986.
6. Lundstrom U, Bull C, Wyse RKH, et al: The natural and "unnatural" history of congenitally corrected transposition. *Am J Cardiol* 65:1222–1229, 1990.

7. Trusler GA, Gonzales JC, Craig BG, et al: Isolated transposition of the great arteries: The present unnatural history, in Doyle EF, Engle MA, Gersony WM, et al (eds): *Paediatric Cardiology*. New York, Springer-Verlag, 1986, pp 1315–1319.

8. Mee RBB: Severe right ventricular failure after Mustard or Senning operation: Two-stage repair. *J Thorac Cardiovasc Surg* 92:385–390, 1986.

9. Graham TP, Atwood GF, Boucek RJ, et al: Abnormalities of right ventricular function following Mustard's operation for transposition of the great arteries. *Circulation* 52:678–684, 1975.

10. Godman MJ, Friedli B, Pasternac A, et al: Hemodynamic studies in children four to ten years after the Mustard operation for transposition of the great arteries. *Circulation* 53:532–538, 1976.

11. Hagler DJ, Ritter DG, Mair DD, et al: Right and left ventricular function after the Mustard procedure in transposition of the great arteries. *Am J Cardiol* 44:276–283, 1979.

12. Parrish MD, Graham TP, Bender HW, et al: Radionuclide angiographic evaluation of right and left ventricular function during exercise after repair of transposition of the great arteries: Comparison with normal subjects and patients with congenitally corrected transposition. *Circulation* 67:178–183, 1983.

13. Benson LN, Bonet J, McLaughlin P, et al: Assessment of right ventricular function during supine bicycle exercise after Mustard's operation. *Circulation* 65:1052–1059, 1982.

14. Ramsay JM, Venables AW, Kelly MJ, et al: RIght and left ventricular function at rest and with exercise after the Mustard operation for transposition of the great arteries. *Br Heart J* 51:364–370, 1984.

15. Graham TP, Jarmakani JM, Atwood GF, et al: Right ventricular volume determinations in children: Normal values and observations with volume or pressure load. *Circulation* 47:144–153, 1973.

16. Graham TP, Jarmakani JM, Canent RV: Left heart volume estimation in infancy and children: Reevaluation of methodology and normal values. *Circulation* 43: 895–904, 1971.

17. Nakazawa M, Marks RA, Isabel-Jones J, et al: Right and left ventricular volume characteristics in children with pulmonary stenosis and intact ventricular septum. *Circulation* 53:884–890, 1976.

18. Nakata S, Imai Y, Takanashi Y, et al: A new method for the quantitative standardization of cross-sectional areas of the pulmonary arteries in congenital heart disease with decreased pulmonary blood flow. *J Thorac Cardiovasc Surg* 88:610–619, 1984.

19. Harada Y, Kawada M, Ishihara K, et al: A new valved conduit with commissures using a glutaraldehyde preserved equine pericardium. *Kyobu Geka* (Japanese text) 42:457–459, 1989.

20. Ilbawi MN, DeLeon SY, Backer CL, et al: An alternative approach to the surgical management for physiologically corrected transposition with ventricular septal defect and pulmonary stenosis or atresia. *J Thorac Cardiovasc Surg* 100:410–411, 1990.

21. Di Donato R, Troconis C, Marino B, et al: Combined Mustard and Rastelli operations: An alternative approach for repair of associated anomalies in congenitally corrected transposition in situs inversus (IDD). *J Thorac Cardiovasc Surg* 104:1246–1248, 1992.

22. Imai Y, Sawatari K, Hoshino S, et al: Ventricular function after anatomical repair in patients with atrioventricular discordance. *J Thorac Cardiovasc Surg* 107:1272–1283, 1994.

23. Lecompte Y, Zannini L, Hanzan E, et al: Anatomic correction of transposition of the great arteries: A new technique without use of a prosthetic conduit. *J Thorac Cardiovasc Surg* 82:629–631, 1981.

24. Anderson KR, Danielson GK, McGoon D, et al: Ebstein's anomaly of the left-sided tricuspid valve: Pathological anatomy of the valvular malformation. *Circulation* 58:87s–91s, 1987.

25. Allwork SP, Bentall HH, Cameron H, et al: Congenitally corrected transposition of the great arteries: Morphologic study of 32 cases. *Am J Cardiol* 38:910–923, 1976.

26. Westerman GR, Lang P, Castaneda AR, et al: Corrected transposition and repair of associated intracardiac defects. *Circulation* 66:197S–202S, 1982.

27. Okamura K, Konno S: Two types of ventricular septal defect in corrected transposition of the great arteries: Reference to surgical approaches. *Am Heart J* 85:483–490, 1973.

28. Anderson RH, Becker AE, Arnold R, et al: The conducting tissue in congenitally corrected transposition. *Circulation* 50:911, 1974.

29. Dick M, Van Praegh R, Rudd M, et al: Electrophysiologic delineation of the specialized atrioventricular conduction system in two patients with corrected transposition of the great arteries in situs inversus (I,D,D). *Circulation* 55:896–900, 1977.

30. Thiene G, Nava A, Rossi L: The conduction system in corrected transposition with situs inversus. *Eur J Cardiol* 6:57–70, 1977.

CHAPTER 5

Volume Reduction Surgery in the Treatment of End-stage Heart Diseases

Tomas A. Salerno, M.D.
Professor of Surgery, Chief of Cardiothoracic Surgery, Division of
Cardiothoracic Surgery, Buffalo General Hospital and State University of
New York at Buffalo, Buffalo, New York

Joginder Bhayana, M.D.
Associate Professor of Surgery, Division of Cardiothoracic Surgery,
Buffalo General Hospital and State University of New York at Buffalo,
Buffalo, New York

Mortality in patients with dilated cardiomyopathy and severe congestive heart failure remains high and is in the range of 40% annually.[1] Orthotopic cardiac transplantation is the main treatment for selected candidates,[2] although it is limited by the number of donor hearts available. Alternative surgical treatments include cardiomyoplasty and left ventricular assist devices (LVADs) as a bridge to transplantation. Until recently, little was available in terms of surgical therapy for patients who are not transplant candidates, especially those with severe dilated cardiomyopathy with or without valvular involvement.

Batista et al.[3] recently introduced a rather bold and innovative procedure, called partial left ventriculectomy, used in the treatment of patients with severe dilated cardiomyopathy. Although controversial, the Batista operation appears to be suitable for all patients with cardiomyopathy, irrespective of age, valvular disease, and etiology of the disease. We will review the principles underlying the Batista operation, describe operative details, postoperative care, current results, and pitfalls, and review the current literature.

Advances in Cardiac Surgery®, vol. 9
© 1997, Mosby–Year Book, Inc.

87

CONCEPTUAL FRAMEWORK

Faced with large numbers of patients with dilated cardiomyopathy of varying etiologies in the south of Brazil, and having made observations in hearts of different species, including humans, Batista empirically concluded that a constant relationship existed between mass (M) and radius (R) in all hearts that he examined. He expressed this relationship as follows: $M = 4 \times R^3$, where R = radius. He then proposed that dilated hearts could be functionally improved if their diameters were reduced (LaPlace's law). In sheep on cardiopulmonary bypass (CPB), Batista performed a left ventriculotomy and closed it by suturing a baffle of bovine pericardium, to simulate left ventricular (LV) dilatation. Immediate deterioration in LV function occurred, which was reversed to control levels when the baffle was removed and the ventriculotomy was closed primarily. Batista had already operated on patients with dilated hearts, by excising a large wedge of LV muscle in an area between the diagonal and posterior descending coronary artery, thereby removing the obtuse marginal branch of the circumflex coronary artery. In some cases, he excised both papillary muscles and mitral valve apparatus to increase the volume of muscle resected and effectively reduce LV diameter. This becomes necessary when the distance between the two papillary muscles is small. Batista reported an operative mortality of 5%, in-hospital mortality of 25%, and 1-year survival of 65%.[4] These results are comparable to those obtained with cardiac transplantation in Brazil. Complete follow-up of his patients is not available because the majority of them are poor and travel long distances from the interior of the country.

At present, little is known about the basic physiology of the Batista operation. It appears that LaPlace's law is the physiologic mechanism involved, i.e., wall tension increases as the heart dilates and decreases when the diameter is reduced. Other mechanisms may be operative, such as humoral factors, peripheral vascular effects, and LV remodeling. Because this is a new procedure, little is known about these mechanisms.

OPERATIVE DETAILS

The principles of surgery outlined herein are as described by Batista. Some surgeons have already modified the operation by using cardioplegic arrest during resection of the ventricle and using different techniques for closure of the ventriculotomy.

After induction of general anesthesia, a transesophageal echocardiography (TEE) probe is inserted to assess valvular competency, cardiac wall motion, and to aid in selecting the area of the left ventricle to be resected. Transesophageal echocardiography is invaluable at the time of weaning from CPB to ensure complete evacuation of cavitary air, to assess segmental wall motion, valvular function, and ejection fraction and volume loading of the ventricles.

Standard cannulation via the ascending aorta and single double-stage venous cannula are usually used. In cases in which tricuspid repair is needed, both cavae are cannulated. Normothermic CPB is instituted and the entire procedure is performed on a beating heart, without aortic clamping or cardioplegia. When cardiac arrest is needed for technical details or safety, increments of 5 mEq of potassium are injected directly into the unclamped ascending aorta, thereby allowing for temporary cardiac standstill. The same amount of potassium chloride (KCl) is injected when ventricular fibrillation occurs during manipulation of the heart, or the heart can be defibrillated via D/C current and internal pads. When tricuspid repair is needed, this is performed at this stage of the procedure. After repair of the valve, the atriotomy is closed and the cavae are unsnared. The left ventricle is then inspected. An injection of 10 mEq of KCl into the ascending aorta arrests the heart before performing the left ventriculotomy incision. The left atrial appendage is opened, and a vent catheter is placed into the left atrial cavity. An incision is made in the apex of the left ventricle at an angle of 45 degrees to the left anterior descending (LAD) coronary artery. The incision is continued into an area between the diagonal and the posterior descending coronary artery. The tip of the scissors is curved away from the septum to prevent deviation of the ventriculectomy incision. Resection of the LV myocardium is carried out by inspection of the internal anatomical landmarks of the ventricle, such as the anterior and posterior papillary muscles, rather than by surface anatomy of the heart. Anomalous chordae are preserved if possible. The incision is carried down to 2 cm from the mitral annulus in an area between both papillary muscles. A wedge of LV myocardium is removed by initiating a second incision at the apex of the ventricle and carrying it posteriorly and laterally, avoiding the posterior papillary muscle. If the papillary muscles are far apart, a large wedge of muscle is excised and the mitral valve apparatus is preserved. Otherwise, the papillary muscles and mitral valve apparatus are removed and the valve is replaced with a prosthesis. The same is the case when mitral valve replacement is planned. Either a mechanical or tissue prosthesis can be used, depending on the clinical situation. In cases of mild mitral regurgitation, valvular repair is performed using the technique described by Fucci et al.[5] This is accomplished by placement of a 4-0 prolene suture at the center of the mitral leaflets, effectively creating a double orifice of the mitral valve.

Details of performance of the ventriculectomy are important, and Batista favors cutting the LV wall in a slightly beveled fashion so that the muscle apposes better during closure. During performance of the ventriculectomy, bleeding coronary vessels are cauterized to prevent inadequate distribution of blood flow in transected vessels. The ventriculectomy is closed with a 2-0 running prolene suture without pledgets, incorporating full thickness of the myocardium, aligning the papillary muscles, and suspending accessory chordae that may have been cut. A 3-0 prolene hemostatic suture is used next to complete closure of the ventriculectomy. Air is removed from the apex of the ventricle after multiple de-airing maneuvers. As mentioned, Batista does not use pledgeted sutures which, he believes, may cause tissue reaction. In some cases, resourcine glue has been used together with a pericardial patch, sutured around the ventriculectomy to control bleeding. When the right ventricle is dilated, as determined intraoperatively by visual inspection or TEE, plicature of the right ventricle is performed. This is done by grasping the free edge of the right ventricle in the redundant area, and suturing it with an over-and-over 2-0 prolene suture from apex to 2 cm from the outflow tract. The suture line is 2 cm from the septum to avoid interference with blood supply to that region.

Before weaning from CPB, nitroprusside is infused to maintain the systolic blood pressure between 90 and 110 mm Hg. This regimen is continued for the first 48 hours to decrease afterload and to prevent hypertension with the risk of bleeding. Inotropes are avoided if possible. An intra-aortic balloon pump (IABP) is invaluable in unstable patients.

An important part of the procedure is identification of the area of muscle to be resected. Evaluation of segmental wall motion by TEE is helpful and, depending on the TEE findings as well as inspection of the surface of the heart and of the open ventricle, the appropriate area of the left ventricle is resected. Coronary artery bypass grafting is usually performed in stenotic vessels unless that area is resected with the vessel, such as an obtuse marginal branch of the circumflex. In cases of cardiomyopathy caused by aortic valvular disease, the aortic valve is replaced first under conditions of cardioplegic arrest. The aorta is then unclamped, and the ventriculectomy is performed in a beating heart. Retrograde cardioplegia cannot be relied on for myocardial protection during ventriculec-tomy because coronary veins are cut. Retrograde perfusion may not deliver adequate flow to the myocardium under these conditions.

The postoperative care of these patients is as in LV aneurysm resection, with particular attention to blood pressure monitoring, the use of vasodilators (nitroprusside), and avoidance of inotropic support. At the time of extubation, hypertension must be avoided because it may cause severe bleeding at the ventriculectomy site. A femoral line, placed during the operation, aids in the insertion of an IABP if necessary.

INDICATIONS FOR THE BATISTA OPERATION

The main indication for the Batista operation is dilated cardiomy-opathy of any etiology. The larger the left ventricle and the lower the ejection fraction (EF), the better the result, according to Batista. The procedure, at least in North America, should be performed electively, because results of emergency surgery have been uni-formly poor in our experience. We believe that in emergency situ-ations, an LVAD should be used and, when stabilized, the patient should be placed on the transplantation list. Alternatively, the heart can be supported for 6 months and then have the assist de-vice removed and a Batista procedure performed, as described by Frazier of the Texas Heart Institute (personal communication, 1996).

CURRENT CLINICAL RESULTS

From 1984 to 1996, Batista described 410 patients with complex cardiac diseases and congestive heart failure.[4] The EF varied from 5% to 18%. Pathologic causes were idiopathic (30%), valvular (20%), ischemic (20%), Chagas' disease (15%), myocarditis (10%), and other (5%). The intraoperative mortality rate was 5%, and the in-hospital mortality rate was 15%. The 1-year survival was 65%. The EF postoperatively increased from 100% to 300%. Complica-tions include renal failure (29 patients), pulmonary embolus (12 patients), and heart failure (9 patients). Bleeding occurred in 6 pa-tients and infection in 4 patients.

Filho et al.[6] described 15 patients with end-stage heart diseases who underwent the Batista operation from December 1994 to De-cember 1995. Survival was 80% at 1 month, 66% at 3 months, 53% at 6 months, 47% at 9 months, and 40% at 12 months. The only detected increment for mortality was associated tricuspid regurgi-tation, which had a death rate of 85%, compared with a death rate of 50% when tricuspid regurgitation was not present. They also found that the Batista operation improved the quality of life of most patients, acting as a bridge to cardiac transplantation when donors are not available. However, sudden death accounted for 58% of the mortality, indicating that arrhythmia is still a major problem after surgery. Unexpectedly, two patients with pulmonary hypertension had decreased pulmonary vascular resistance after the Batista operation. A similar experience was reported by Lucchese et al.[7] in 2 of 20 patients who had a decrease in pulmonary vascular resistance after the Batista operation.

Angelini[8] described 14 patients from June 1995 to February 1996 who underwent the Batista operation in three international centers. All had an EF less than 20%, and the etiology of their diseases was idiopathic (6 patients), ischemic (5 patients), and valvular (3 patients). One death occurred in the operating room. Two additional deaths occurred on the third and seventh postoperative day because of heart failure. One patient died of hemorrhage on the first postoperative day. Two late deaths at 11 and 12 weeks resulted from biventricular failure. Of the 8 survivors, 3 patients are in New York Heart Association (NYHA) class I and 5 are in class II.

Stolf et al.[9] described 21 patients with congestive heart failure and dilated cardiomyopathy who underwent volume reduction surgery and were in NYHA class III and IV. There were 3 hospital deaths (15%). The LV diameter decreased from 81.3 ± 9.6 mm to 68.3 ± 9.1 mm ($P < 0.001$), and LV wall shortening from 11.1 ± 3.2 mm to 15.4 ± 2.9 mm ($P < 0.04$). Four patients died at midterm follow-up because of congestive heart failure (1 patient) and arrhythmia (3 patients). The actuarial survival was $62.3 \pm 11.3\%$ at 12 months, with NYHA class improvement from 3.2 ± 0.8 to 1.4 ± 0.6.

Bombanato et al.[10] operated on 10 patients from February to June 1995. All patients were in NYHA class IV. Three patients were receiving inotropic support, large doses of diuretics, vasodilators, and digitalis. Left ventricular dimensions were 78.29 ± 12.63 mm, and the EF was 0.15 ± 0.05. There was no mortality in this series of patients. Functional class improved to 1.71 ± 0.48 NYHA ($P = 0.009$), LV dimension to 64.67 ± 11.41 mm ($P = 0.02$), and EF to 0.22 ± 0.04 ($P = 0.02$).

The Buffalo General Hospital was the first center outside Brazil to perform the Batista operation. The first patient, a 56-year-old architect with cardiomyopathy, had sustained two myocardial infarctions, had a history of pulmonary edema, and was severely symptomatic. He was given a choice of going on the transplantation list or undergoing this experimental procedure, which had just been approved by our institutional review board committee. With informed consent, he underwent partial left ventriculectomy on July 24, 1995. He left the hospital 15 days after uncomplicated surgery and has resumed a normal life. One month after surgery he was playing golf, sailing, and hunting. He continues to do well at this time. Since then, we have performed 18 partial ventriculectomies. Ten of these patients are alive at present. Most of the deaths resulted from case selection, because our IRB document recommended only those patients who were not transplantation candidates. Therefore, patients operated on were elderly, some were extremely ill with multiorgan diseases, or those who refused transplantation for one reason or another. At this time we pay particular attention to the indications for surgery and case selection, avoiding ischemic heart diseases and patients who have had multiple procedures. We have initiated an international registry of the Batista operation to fully accumulate worlwide experience and to delineate the benefits of this procedure. As we gain more experience with this procedure, especially regarding the indications for surgery, it is expected that mortality will decrease. Some of the early and late deaths are caused by arrhythmias, and this may be decreased by appropriate electrophysiologic (EP) studies, drugs such as amiodarone, and implantation of defibrillators.

PITFALLS

The Batista operation has generated great enthusiasm among cardiac surgeons and, in our view, represents an important development in cardiac surgery. There are many questions that need to be clarified, such as indications and timing of surgery, long-term results, and potential for redilatation. Issues such as the need for cardioplegic arrest and the type of ventriculectomy closure to ensure safety and prevent bleeding are being addressed. Assessment of left ventricular stroke work, wall tension, remodeling, and mechanisms of action are currently being investigated.

Surgeons should be cautioned that considerable skills and judgment are needed in performing this operation. This is not simply an LV aneurysm resection procedure. At time of surgery, global hypokinesia with no discrete area to be resected is usually found. As a word of caution, it is advisable to await results from centers currently performing this procedure. Only then will we be in a position to recommend the Batista operation for widespread use. At present, it is recommended that centers with the capability of transplantation and/or long-term LV assistance be involved in performing the Batista operation. Furthermore, surgeons are encouraged to visit a colleague or center that is performing the procedure to become familiar with the details of the surgery.

The perioperative management is of great importance in the Batista operation. Anesthesiologists and surgeons are accustomed to dealing with seriously ill patients, and inotropic support is usually used. In the Batista operation, initially only nitroprusside is used. In some cases in our experience, it was required to insert IABP (which we use now liberally), and use inotropic support in somes cases. Furthermore, it is important to maintain the patients on their respective regimens of medication postoperatively and make the necessary adjustments slowly. Atrial fibrillation must be treated aggressively because patients tolerate it poorly. Because of the decreased size of the heart and the large pericardial sac after surgery, pericardial effusion is a problem. Batista recommends leaving the pericardial chest tubes for 3 days or until the return is clear. Bleeding perioperatively can be troublesome, and some deaths have been attributed to bleeding at the suture line. One frustrating aspect of this procedure is that some patients have spectacular results from surgery with EF increasing from 12% to 50%, whereas other patients do not seem to improve. Perhaps preoperative biopsy may aid in identifying those patients who will not improve. Frazier from the Texas Heart Institute has removed LVAD and performed the Batista procedure. Patients were weaned from the device when the ventricle was made smaller by the Batista procedure (personal communication, 1996). Although this experience is limited, it has opened up new avenues to treat patients with dilated cardiomyopathy.

How should the Batista operation be viewed at this time? As a new procedure, the Batista operation should be considered experimental. As such, we recommend that institutional review board approval and informed consent be obtained in patients being offered this procedure. We suggest that centers planning to perform the Batista operation have an LVAD at their disposal. Heart transplantation should be available to young patients should the operation fail acutely or in the long-term. Careful follow-up of these patients is essential to fully delineate the effects of this procedure. An international registry of these patients is being organized at the State University of New York at Buffalo in collaboration with other centers worlwide.

SUMMARY

Originated in South America, the Batista operation offers a new option in the treatment of patients with end-stage heart diseases. The procedure, in its infancy, appears to be beneficial to patients with severe dilated cardiomyopathy. Indications for surgery are evolving, and long-term results are not available presently. Surgeons interested in this procedure should gain experience from other centers performing the surgery. We recommend that institutional review board approval and informed consent be obtained from patients who are to undergo this procedure.

REFERENCES

1. Consensus Investigators: Effects of enalapril on mortality in severe congestive heart failure. *N Engl J Med* 316:1429–1435, 1987.
2. Kriett JM, Kaye MP: The registry of International Society of Heart and Lung Transplantation: Eighth official report: 1991. *J Heart Lung Transplant* 10:491–498, 1991.
3. Batista JV, Santos JLV, Takeshita N, et al: Partial left ventriculectomy to improve left ventricular function in end-stage heart disease. *J Cardiac Surg* 11:96–97, 1996.
4. Batista JV, Santos JVL, Cunha MA, et al: Ventriculectomia parcial: Um novo conceito no tratamento cirurgico de cardiopatias em fase final. Anais do XXII Congresso Nacional de Cirurgia Cardiaca, Brasilia. Sociedade Brasileira de Cirurgia Cardiaca, 1995, pp 150–151.
5. Fucci C, Sandrelli B, Pardini A, et al: Improved results with mitral valve repair using new surgical techniques. *Eur J Cardiothorac Surg* 9:621–627, 1995.
6. Filho F, Pereira WM, Leases PE, et al: End-stage heart disease: Is there a role for Batista operation? Presented at International Meeting: Surgical Options for End-Stage Heart Failure. Bergamo, Italy, Sept 14, 1996.
7. Lucchese FA, Filho FJD, Pereira WM, et al: Initial experience with the Batista's partial left ventriculectomy. Annual Congress of the Cardiovascular Society of the State of Rio Grande do Sul, Brazil, October 1995.
8. Angelini GD: Left ventricular volume reduction for end-stage heart disease: Preliminary clinical results and proposal of an international multicenter registry and prospective study. Presented at International Meeting: Surgical Options for End-Stage Heart Failure. Bergamo, Italy, Sept 14, 1996.
9. Stolf NAG, Moreira LFP, Bocchi EAB, et al: Early results of reductive left ventriculoplasty in the treatment of dilated cardiomyopathy. Presented at International Meeting: Surgical Options for End-Stage Heart Failure. Bergamo, Italy, Sept 14, 1996.
10. Bombanato R, Bestelli RB, Sgarbieri R, et al: Initial experience with Batista's partial left ventriculectomy for the treatment of terminal and refractory heart failure. *Arq Bras Cardiol* 66:189–192, 1996.

CHAPTER 6

Video-assisted Coronary Surgery

Guido Sani, M.D.
Istituto di Chirurgia Toracica e Cardiovascolare, Università di Siena,
Siena, Italy

Gianfranco Lisi, M.D.
Istituto di Chirurgia Toracica e Cardiovascolare, Università di Siena,
Siena, Italy

Massimo A. Mariani, M.D.
Istituto di Chirurgia Toracica e Cardiovascolare, Università di Siena,
Siena, Italy

Massimo Maccherini, M.D.
Istituto di Chirurgia Toracica e Cardiovascolare, Università di Siena,
Siena, Italy

Patrick Nataf, M.D.
Service de Chirurgie Cardiaque, Hôpital de la Pitié, Paris, France

Federico J. Benetti, M.D.
Fundaciòn Benetti, Buenos Aires, Argentina

Michele Toscano, M.D.
Istituto di Chirurgia Toracica e Cardiovascolare, Università di Siena,
Siena, Italy

C oronary artery bypass grafting (CABG) is an established technique for the treatment of coronary artery disease and is the most frequently performed surgical procedure in the industrialized countries. Continuous refinements in surgical technique, in myocardial protection, and in intraoperative and postoperative management have improved the results of CABG but have caused a general rise in cost of medical care.[1]

In-hospital mortality and morbidity seem to have reached a plateau in terms of results because of the concurrence of two opposing factors: (1) the aforementioned technical refinements, and (2) the general tendency to accept an increasing number of high-risk patients.[2] The increasing number of high-risk patients has further raised the cost of medical care, because of the increased in-hospital morbidity. Therefore, researchers are now investigating alternative methods of surgical myocardial revascularization to improve the results of CABG while reducing the cost of medical care.

The reduction of systemic inflammatory response[3] is a promising field of research for the improvement of the results in CABG. The reduction of systemic inflammatory response can lead to a reduction of in-hospital morbidity and mortality.[4] The avoidance of cardiopulmonary bypass (CPB)[5] and the reduction of surgical impact appear to be the most effective means to decrease the systemic inflammatory response after CABG. In fact, the wound has proven to be an incremental determinant of systemic inflammatory response in CABG.[6] However, the avoidance of CPB and the use of a small surgical access undoubtedly increase the technical difficulty of coronary surgery because of the absence of a restless and bloodless operative field. Moreover, the cardiovascular structures are viewed from a different and unusual angle through a small surgical access.

Therefore, the acceptance of minimally invasive CABG (MICABG) is subordinate to the achievement of the same results as obtained with conventional coronary surgery. In this respect, video-assisting devices can offer concrete help.

LESS INVASIVE CORONARY SURGERY: CORONARY ARTERY BYPASS GRAFTING WITHOUT CARDIOPULMONARY BYPASS

The first pioneering experiences with CABG without CPB were made at the beginning of the 1970s[7, 8] and were not followed by a general acceptance. In the next phase, during the 1980s, Buffolo et al. and Benetti et al. reported the first large series of patients who successfully underwent CABG without CPB.[9, 10] These large experiences led to a renewed worldwide interest in CABG without CPB at the beginning of the 1990s. We adopted this technique in the Department of Cardiothoracic Surgery of Siena at the end of 1994. Since then we have performed more than 200 CABG procedures without CPB via midline sternotomy and have found that the anastomosis on the left anterior descending (LAD) and right coronary artery (RCA) is feasible, whereas the anastomosis on marginal branches is technically more challenging for the surgeon and hemodynamically less tolerated.

The advantages of CABG without CPB seem more evident for high-risk patients. We operated on 40 high-risk patients[11] who had one or more of the following risk factors: postischemic cardiomyopathy, extensive aortic calcification, cerebrovascular disease or carotid stenoses, and chronic renal insufficiency. In these patients, neither operative death nor noncardiac complication (cerebrovascular accidents, kidney failure, prolonged ventilatory support, sepsis) occurred; conversely, a perioperative myocardial infarction occurred in 7 patients (14.2%), 1 of whom needed intra-aortic counterpulsation. The mean postoperative hospital stay was 6.3 ± 3.2 days. The short postoperative hospital stay of these high-risk patients was favored by the absence of noncardiac complications. However, the rate of early recurrence of angina (7.7%) reported by Moshkovitz et al. in 220 patients operated on without CPB[12] suggests the need for further technical improvement in the anastomosis performed without CPB to achieve the same accuracy and reliability as with conventional coronary surgery.

MINIMALLY INVASIVE CORONARY ARTERY BYPASS GRAFTING

A further evolution in the concept of CABG without CPB was the introduction of MICABG by Benetti et al. in 1994.[13] Minimally invasive CABG is a radically new approach to surgical myocardial revascularization and is performed through a small anterolateral thoracotomy without CPB. Thus, MICABG combines two advantages: a small surgical access and the avoidance of CPB. Minimally invasive CABG enables the surgeon to anastomose the left or the right internal mammary artery (IMA) to the LAD or the RCA, respectively.

In the original description of MICABG made by Benetti et al., the surgical access was performed through a 4- to 10-cm anterolateral thoracotomy in the fifth intercostal space. The left IMA was then harvested from the origin until the sixth intercostal space, with the aid of a video-thoracoscope. The thoracoscope was inserted in the sixth intercostal space along the anterior axillary line and was used to facilitate the harvesting of the proximal part of the left IMA. The instruments for harvesting the IMA and for performing the left IMA-to-LAD anastomosis were inserted through the small anterolateral thoracotomy.

After the original description of MICABG, a few different variations of the original technique have been published (Table 1). As for the early results of MICABG (Table 2), these different techniques had two characteristics in common: the small number of cases and the initial learning curve, which led to the conversion to midline sternotomy and CPB in some cases. In addition, the reported rate of perioperative myocardial infarction was higher than expected,

TABLE 1.

Methods of Minimally Invasive Coronary Artery Bypass Grafting

Reference	Surgical Approach	IMA Harvesting	VTS	CPB
Benetti et al.[13]	Minithoracotomy	Complete	Yes*	No
Robinson et al.[14]	Parasternal	Complete	Yes*	Yes
Arom et al.[15]	Ministernotomy	Complete	No	No
Stanbridge et al.[16]	Parasternal	Incomplete	No	No
Calafiore et al.[17]	Minithoracotomy	Incomplete	No	No
Nataf et al.[18]	Minithoracotomy	Complete	Yes†	No
Acuff et al.[19]	Minithoracotomy	Complete	Yes†	No

*Video-thoracoscopy–aided harvesting of IMA through minithoracotomy.
†Video-thoracoscopic harvesting of IMA before minithoracotomy.
Abbreviations: IMA, internal mammary artery; *VTS,* video-thoracoscopy; *CPB,* cardiopulmonary bypass.

TABLE 2.

Early Results and Pitfalls of Minimally Invasive Coronary Artery Bypass Grafting

Reference	*n*	POMI	POM	Conversion*	Graft Patency
Nataf et al.[18]	20	0%	0%	5%	86.6%
Alessandrini et al.[21]	32	6.2%	3.1%	3.1%	—
Mack[22]	20	0%	0%	10%	—
Calafiore et al.[17]	162	4.5%	0.6%	4.3%	95.5%†
Boonstra[23]	50	4%	0%	4.4%	—
Stanbridge et al.[16]	25	0%	0%	0%	93.6%
Jansen[24]	13	0%	0%	0%	86.7%

*Need of conversion to sternotomy.
†Doppler evaluation in most cases.
Abbreviations: POMI, postoperative myocardial infarction; *POM,* postoperative mortality.

and the patency of the IMA at early angiographic control did not reach 100%. In Table 3, the problems that we and other authors have encountered during MICABG procedures, which have led to these partially unsatisfactory results, are summarized. These problems seemed to result from the three basic steps of the MICABG: harvesting of the IMA, identification of the target coronary vessel, and mammary-to-coronary anastomosis.

TABLE 3.
Problems Encountered During the First Minimally Invasive Coronary
Artery Bypass Grafting *(MICABG)* Experiences

Problems of MICABG related to the IMA:
1. increased difficulty in harvesting the IMA (lesions of the IMA,
   length of the IMA pedicle, stretching of the minithoracotomy)
2. IMA pedicle too short to reach the chosen site of anastomosis
   (kinking of the IMA pedicle, tension on the anastomosis)

Problems of MICABG related to the coronary vessel:
1. identifying the vessel (intramyocardial vessel, mistaken vessel)
2. performing the anastomosis at the optimal site of the target
   coronary vessel (a short IMA pedicle might not reach the optimal
   site)

Problems of MICABG related to the anastomosis:
1. difficult handling of tissues as a result of the motion of the target
   coronary vessel
2. bleeding operative field (limited vision)

Abbreviation: IMA, internal mammary artery.

HARVESTING OF THE INTERNAL MAMMARY ARTERY

The basic principle is that the IMA pedicle must be harvested from
its origin down to the sixth intercostal space, similar to the way
this is done via midline sternotomy. The reasons for such a principle are both theoretical and practical. Theoretically, applying the
same technique as the one used in midline sternotomy, MICABG
will benefit from the long-term angiographic studies on the IMA
patency already carried out in the past two decades. Therefore, a
long-term angiographic follow-up will not be necessary. In addition, there will be no need to investigate whether the effect of the
"steal" from side branches is really negligible. A long pedicle also
allows the surgeon to choose the best site for the anastomosis on
the diseased coronary vessel.

Video-thoracoscopy can be extremely useful for obtaining a
completely free IMA pedicle. Practically, a long IMA pedicle
avoids kinking and tension on the mammary-to-coronary anastomosis that leads to catastrophic consequences. In particular, the
video-thoracoscopic harvesting of the IMA allows a minimal thoracotomy and avoids the excessive stretch of the wound or the excision of cartilage—usually necessary for a direct-view IMA harvesting—which may cause increased postoperative pain. Other
techniques may provide a shorter IMA pedicle. In fact, Calafiore

and colleagues[20] described the need to elongate the IMA with an inferior epigastric artery graft in 25 of 240 cases. In our opinion, harvesting of IMA should be video-thoracoscopic and should be carried out before performing the minithoracotomy, by means of three separate chest ports in which the thoracoscope and two grasping or cutting instruments (electrocauthery or scissors) are inserted. In his experience of 20 uncomplicated cases, Nataf et al.[18] suggest making the chest ports in the fourth and sixth intercostal space along the median axillary line and in the fifth intercostal space along the anterior axillary line. Conversely, Acuff et al.[19] suggest making the chest ports in the third, fourth, and fifth intercostal space along the posterior axillary line.

The complete thoracoscopic harvesting of the IMA is undoubtedly a challenging issue, especially for cardiac surgeons who are not familiar with thoracoscopy. However, thoracoscopic instruments especially developed for IMA harvesting are now becoming available. In particular, thoracoscopic electrocautheries with a built-in irrigation-suction device and thoracoscopic ultrasound cautheries[25] have been recently introduced into clinical use.

Another interesting aspect of the video-thoracoscopic harvesting of the IMA is the visualization of the operative images. Traditional video-assisting devices display images on a video monitor. Thus, the surgeon must constantly maintain visual contact with the monitor. Turning away the head from the monitor causes the surgeon to lose control of the surgical site. Recently, head-mounted displays have been developed for thoracoscopic use.[26] These devices enable the surgeon to see the operative field as well as the surgical site at the same time. Furthermore, head-mounted displays can now produce a three-dimensional view by means of stereoscopic pictures made of two fields. Head-mounted three-dimensional displays will certainly change the "point of view" of many cardiac surgeons with respect to MICABG.

IDENTIFICATION OF THE TARGET CORONARY VESSEL

Identification of the target coronary vessel is one of the most frequently encountered problems in cases of conversion of MICABG to midline sternotomy. This problem can be circumvented by an IMA pedicle that is long enough to enable the surgeon to choose the best site for the anastomosis. Video-thoracoscopic devices can also be helpful in identifying the target coronary vessel before performing the thoracotomy, with a preliminary video-thoracoscopic intrapericardial inspection.

MAMMARY-TO-CORONARY ANASTOMOSIS

The target of the MICABG is a technically perfect mammary-to-coronary anastomosis. However, the mammary-to-coronary anastomosis on the beating heart without CPB and by means of a small anterolateral thoracotomy is technically more demanding than the anastomosis on the arrested heart. Therefore one of the main fields of research in MICABG is the method of stabilization of the target coronary vessel during the anastomosis. The methods of stabilization can be mechanical or pharmacologic.

Various methods of mechanical stabilization are under consideration, and two are currently available: the CTS Stabilizer (Stabilizer, CardioThoracic System, Cupertino, Calif.)[27] and the Octopus.[28] Mechanical coronary stabilizers are designed to reduce the movements of the target coronary vessel during the anastomosis, without affecting the hemodynamics. The two looping sutures, normally used to occlude the coronary vessel, reduce the movements only on the horizontal plane (X,Y), mainly along the longitudinal axis of the vessel. However, the two looping sutures are less effective in reducing the transverse movements and are null in avoiding the movements on the vertical (Z) plane. The stabilizers, indeed, minimize the vertical movements (Z plane) and contribute to strongly reducing the transverse movements on the horizontal plane.

The pharmacologic stabilization of the heart can be achieved with short-acting β-blockers (esmolol)[29] or with the use of repeated boluses of adenosine (Acuff TE, personal communication). Adenosine can induce brief periods of reversible asystole, thus ensuring a motionless operative field for some seconds.

CONCLUSION

The recent progress and rapid worldwide diffusion of MICABG have triggered a palpable surge of interest in this new technique. Nowadays, MICABG is generally considered complementary to conventional CABG and an alternative to percutaneous transluminal coronary angioplasty in the treatment of single-vessel disease, in particular, the isolated stenosis of the LAD. In selected cases, MICABG can also be offered to patients with two-vessel disease (LAD and circumflex artery). In fact, the anterolateral minithoracotomy provides a good exposure of the lateral wall of the heart. In one patient with two-vessel disease,[30] we performed a complete arterial revascularization with a T-graft of radial artery anastomosed end-to-side to the IMA. The IMA was anastomosed to the

LAD, and the radial artery was anastomosed to the first diagonal branch and the first marginal branch as a sequential graft. A long IMA pedicle was needed to perform an anastomosis without any tension on the arms of the T-graft. However, the adoption of the IMA-to-LAD grafting with MICABG in patients with two- or three-vessel disease is limited.

With MICABG it is obviously not possible to achieve a complete revascularization in patients with two- or three-vessel disease. In these patients, a complete revascularization, as achieved with conventional coronary surgery without CPB, is correlated with better long-term survival and freedom from cardiac adverse events.[31, 32] Therefore, the treatment of the culprit lesion is a strongly controversial issue in our opinion. Minimally invasive CABG is a technically demanding operation, as pointed out after the live teleconference on less invasive coronary bypass surgery held in Oxford in March 1996.[33]

Some of the initial controversial results were mainly caused by the compound effect of the learning curve and the lack of specific instruments. Because the learning curve is an unavoidable variable, the research has focused on the development of specific instruments, and recently a large number of new instruments and devices have become available. Among them video-assisting thoracoscopic devices will play an important role in improving the harvesting of the IMA, as well as in further minimizing the surgical access. Thus, the progress in video-assisting devices has the potential to improve the surgical results and minimize the surgical impact on the patients even more. It is hoped that this will reflect into an improvement of mortality and morbidity in patients with single-vessel disease.

Today, patients with single-vessel disease can be offered MICABG as an alternative treatment that is better tolerated than conventional CABG via midline sternotomy and has better long-term results than percutaneous transluminal coronary angioplasty. Prospective randomized clinical trials comparing percutaneous transluminal coronary angioplasty, MICABG, and conventional CABG via midline sternotomy in patients with single-vessel disease will shed further light on this issue. However, we are convinced that the future of MICABG is strictly correlated to three main factors: patient selection, adequate training in coronary surgery without CPB via midline sternotomy, and improvement of specific instruments and video-assisting devices.

ACKNOWLEDGMENT

We thank H. Los, M.A., for her support in preparing the manuscript.

REFERENCES

1. Hannan EL, Kilburn H Jr, Racz M, et al: Improving the outcomes of coronary artery bypass surgery in New York State. *JAMA* 271:761–766, 1994.
2. Cristakis GT, Ivanov J, Weisel RD, et al: The changing pattern of coronary artery bypass surgery. *Circulation* 80:151S–161S, 1989.
3. Kirklin JK, Westaby S, Blackstone EH, et al: Complement and the damaging effects of cardiopulmonary bypass. *J Thorac Cardiovasc Surg* 86:845–857, 1983.
4. Butler J, Rocker GM, Westaby S: Inflammatory response to cardiopulmonary bypass. *Ann Thorac Surg* 55:552–559, 1993.
5. Edmunds LH: Why cardiopulmonary bypass makes patients sick: Strategies to control the blood–synthetic surface interface, in Karp RB, Laks H, Wechsler AS (eds): *Advances in Cardiac Surgery*, vol 6. St Louis, Mosby, 1995, pp 131–167.
6. de Haan J, Boonstra PW, Tabuchi N, et al: Retransfusion of thoracic wound blood during cardiac surgery obscures biocompatibilty of the extracorporeal circuit. *J Thorac Cardiovasc Surg* 112:275–276, 1996.
7. Ankeney JL: To use or not use the pump oxygenator in coronary bypass operations. *Ann Thorac Surg* 19:108–109, 1975.
8. Trapp WG, Bisarya R: Placement of coronary artery bypass graft without pump oxygenator. *Ann Thorac Surg* 19:1–9, 1975.
9. Buffolo E, Andrade JCS, Branco JNR, et al: Myocardial revascularization without extra-corporeal circulation: Seven year experience in 593 cases. *Eur J Cardiothorac Surg* 4:504–508, 1990.
10. Benetti FJ, Naselli G, Wood M, et al: Direct myocardial revascularization without extracorporeal circulation. Experience in 700 patients. *Chest* 100:312–316, 1991.
11. Sani G, Mariani MA, Lisi G, et al: Coronary artery bypass surgery without cardiopulmonary bypass in high risk patients, in Abstract Book of the *Proceedings of the 1st International Live Teleconference on Least-Invasive Coronary Surgery.* Oxford, March 1996, pp 39–48.
12. Moshkovitz Y, Lusky A, Mohr R: Coronary artery bypass without cardiopulmonary bypass: Analysis of short-term and mid-term outcome in 220 patients. *J Thorac Cardiovasc Surg* 110:979–987, 1995.
13. Benetti FJ, Ballester C, Sani G, et al: Video assisted coronary artery bypass grafting. *J Card Surg* 10:620–625, 1995.
14. Robinson MC, Gross DR, Zeman W, et al.: Minimally invasive coronary artery bypass grafting: A new method using an anterior mediastinotomy. *J Card Surg* 10:529–536, 1995.
15. Arom KV, Emery RW, Nicoloff DM: Mini-sternotomy for coronary artery bypass grafting. *Ann Thorac Surg* 61:1271–1272, 1996.
16. Stanbridge R, Symons GV, Banwell PE: Minimal access surgery for coronary artery revascularisation. *Lancet* 346:837, 1995.
17. Calafiore AM, Di Gianmarco G, Teodori G, et al: Left anterior descending coronary artery grafting via left anterior small thoracotomy without cardiopulmonary bypass. *Ann Thorac Surg* 61:1658–1665, 1996.

18. Nataf P, Lima L, Regan M, et al.: Minimally invasive coronary surgery with thoracoscopic internal mammary artery dissection: Surgical technique. *J Card Surg* 11:288–292, 1997.

19. Acuff TE, Landrenau RJ, Mack MJ, et al.: Minimally invasive coronary artery bypass grafting. *Ann Thorac Surg* 61:135–137, 1996.

20. Calafiore AM, Teodori G, Di Gianmarco G, et al: Inferior epigastric elongation of mammary artery during LAD grafting via a left anterior small thoracotomy, in Abstract Book of the *Proceedings of the 10th Annual Meeting of the European Association for Cardio-Thoracic Surgery.* Prague, October 1996, p 132A.

21. Alessandrini F, Luciani N, Possati GF, et al: Early complication of the minimally invasive thoracotomy for myocardial revascularisation, in Abstract Book of the *Proceedings of the 10th Annual Meeting of the European Association for Cardio-Thoracic Surgery.* Prague, October 1996, p 256.

22. Mack M: Minimally invasive thoracoscopically assisted coronary artery bypass grafting, in Abstract Book of the *Proceedings of the 10th Annual Meeting of the European Association for Cardio-Thoracic Surgery.* Prague, October 1996, p 112.

23. Boonstra PW, Grandjean JG, van Weerd E: Clinical experience with minimally invasive coronary bypass grafting without cardiopulmonary bypass, in Abstract Book of the *Proceedings of the 10th Annual Meeting of the European Association for Cardio-Thoracic Surgery.* Prague, October 1996, p 114.

24. Jansen EWL, Grundeman PF, Borst C, et al: Coronary artery revascularisation on the beating heart using local wall immobilisation: The "Octopus" method via a limited approach, in Abstract Book of the *Proceedings of the 10th Annual Meeting of the European Association for Cardio-Thoracic Surgery.* Prague, October 1996, p 258.

25. Wolf RK, Ohtsuka T, Hiratzka LF, et al: Thoracoscopic IMA harvest for MICABG using the Harmonic Scalpel, in Abstract Book of the *Proceedings of the 2nd Workshop on MICABG.* Utrecht, October 1996, p 12.

26. Pankratov MM, Lonn U, Casimir-Ahn H: 3D or not 3D? The fundamental of 3D surgical visualization, in Abstract Book of the *Proceedings of the 2nd Workshop on MICABG.* Utrecht, October 1996, p 9.

27. Boonstra PW, Grandjean JG, Mariani MA: An improved method for direct coronary grafting without CPB via antero-lateral small thoracotomy. *Ann Thorac Surg,* in press.

28. Borst C, Jansen EW, Bredèe JJ, et al: Coronary artery bypass without cardiopulmonary bypass and without interruption of native coronary flow using a novel anastomosis site restraining device ("Octopus"). *J Am Coll Cardiol* 27:1356–1364, 1996.

29. Labovitz AJ, Barth C, Castello R, et al: Attenuation of myocardial ischemia during coronary occlusion by ultrashort-acting beta adrenergic blockade. *Am Heart J* 121:1347–1352, 1991.

30. Sani G, Benetti FJ, Mariani MA, et al: Arterial myocardial revascularization without cardiopulmonary bypass through a small thoracotomy. *Eur J Cardiothorac Surg* 10:699–701, 1996.

31. Jones EL, Weintraub WS: The importance of completeness of revascularization during long-term follow-up after coronary artery operations. *J Thorac Cardiovasc Surg* 112:227–237, 1996.

32. Sergeant P, Blackstone E, Meyns B, et al: The early and late influence of patient procedural and surgical experience variables on survival after CABG, in Abstract Book of the *Proceedings of the 10th Annual Meeting of the European Association for Cardio-Thoracic Surgery.* Prague, October 1996, p 100.

33. Westaby S, Benetti FJ: Less invasive coronary surgery: Consensus from the Oxford meeting. *Ann Thorac Surg* 62:924–931, 1996.

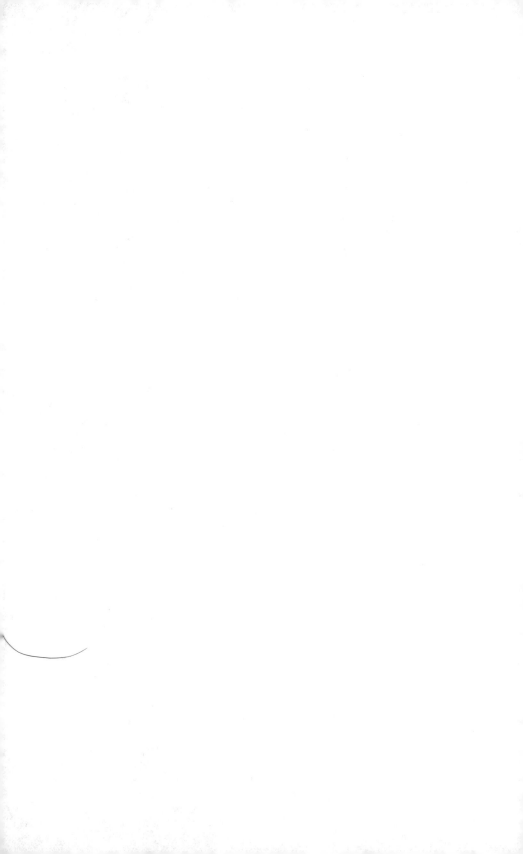

CHAPTER 7

Postoperative Atrial Fibrillation

Kenneth A. Ellenbogen, M.D.
Associate Professor of Medicine, Department of Medicine, Division of Cardiology, Medical College of Virginia and McGuire VA Medical Center, Richmond, Virginia

Mina K. Chung, M.D.
Department of Cardiology, The Cleveland Clinic, Cleveland, Ohio

Craig R. Asher, M.D.
Department of Cardiology, The Cleveland Clinic, Cleveland, Ohio

Mark A. Wood, M.D.
Assistant Professor of Medicine, Department of Medicine, Division of Cardiology, Medical College of Virginia and McGuire VA Medical Center, Richmond, Virginia

A trial fibrillation remains one of the most common postoperative complications of coronary artery bypass grafting (CABG) and valvular surgery. With more than 400,000 open-heart procedures performed yearly in the United States, learning more about the optimal management of atrial fibrillation in the postoperative setting becomes an important goal of clinical research. The increasing mean age of patients undergoing open-heart surgery is expected to result in an increased incidence of postoperative atrial fibrillation and greater costs for the management of these patients. Several recent excellent reviews are recommended for the interested reader.[1, 2]

EPIDEMIOLOGY

Supraventricular arrhythmias are common after all major surgical procedures, including thoracic and abdominal surgical procedures. The incidence of atrial fibrillation and atrial flutter was reported by Favaloro et al. to be 12% in the first 100 patients undergoing CABG at the Cleveland Clinic from 1967 to 1968.[3] The incidence of supraventricular arrhythmias was reported to be 4% by Goldman in a large registry of patients undergoing major noncardiac surgery.[4] A multicenter study of patients undergoing abdominal aortic aneurysm repair reported an incidence of supraventricular arrhythmias of 3.2%, and in a prospective study of 295 patients undergoing thoracotomy for lung cancer, the incidence of supraventricular arrhythmias was almost 13%.[5, 6] Data published during the past decade show an incidence of atrial fibrillation after CABG that varies considerably between studies, ranging from 5% to 40%.[1] A recent preliminary report from the Cleveland Clinic cited an incidence of postoperative atrial fibrillation of 19% in 42 patients undergoing minimally invasive cardiac surgery, which was similar to the incidence of atrial fibrillation for patients undergoing CABG using standard techniques.[7] Two recent prospective multicenter studies of CABG from the 1990s reported an incidence of postoperative atrial fibrillation between 27% and 33%.[8, 9] The incidence of atrial fibrillation is higher in patients undergoing valve replacement with or without CABG, occurring in 30% to 70% of patients.

Atrial fibrillation may occur at any time after CABG, but generally occurs 2–4 days after open-heart surgery.[8, 9] The episodes generally tend to be transient, short-lived, frequent, and recurrent. Atrial fibrillation occurs less commonly immediately (less than 24 hours) or late (greater than 5 days) after bypass surgery with a time course approximating a bell-shaped curve and the peak occurring 2–4 days after surgery (Fig 1). Episodes may recur or persist for weeks before finally resolving spontaneously. Up to 10% to 15% of patients with post-CABG atrial fibrillation are discharged from the hospital with atrial fibrillation. It is rare for chronic atrial fibrillation to develop after CABG.

PATHOPHYSIOLOGY

Multiple mechanisms have been proposed responsible for the pathogenesis of atrial fibrillation in the postoperative setting.[10] These mechanisms include acute atrial distension or inflammation from the trauma of surgery; alteration in autonomic tone from surgery and the stress of the postoperative period; ischemic injury to atria as a result of surgery and/or inadequate protection during bypass; electrolyte and volume shifts during bypass resulting in changes in repolarization; inflammation resulting from pericarditis; and a variety of other electrophysiologic changes that may occur as a result of the bypass procedure, the cardioplegia, or the surgery itself that all may result in a lower atrial fibrillation threshold.

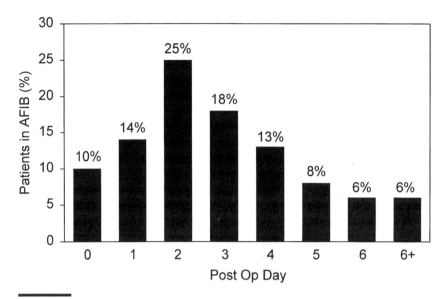

FIGURE 1.

Time of occurrence of atrial fibrillation *(AFIB)* after coronary artery bypass grafting. (Courtesy of Aranki SF, Shaw DP, Adams DH, et al: Predictors of atrial fibrillation after coronary artery surgery. Current trends and impact on hospital resources. *Circulation* 94:390–397. Copyright 1996, American Heart Association. Reproduced with permission.)

The pathophysiology of atrial fibrillation in the nonsurgical setting has been intensively studied. One of the more widely held theories is the multiple wavelet hypothesis advanced by Moe.[11] This theory proposes that atrial fibrillation is the result of multiple wavelets caused by reentry that move through the atria constantly colliding or extinguishing themselves, and reforming or combining with new wavelets. Mapping studies in animals and humans have demonstrated these multiple wavelets, whose course is dictated by atrial conduction, refractoriness, and excitability.[12] The wavelets are believed to be primarily functionally determined, and a predisposition to atrial reentry is caused by a combination of several factors including heterogeneity of conduction in the atria, large atrial size, alterations in electrical coupling in the atrial myocardium, and fixed anatomical obstacles.

The mechanism of postoperative atrial fibrillation is less well defined. Multiple mechanisms likely play a role. Several electrophysiologic changes that may predispose to atrial fibrillation have been documented to occur in the postoperative setting. For example, Chung and colleagues have performed a series of studies before and after bypass showing suppressed sinus node function after CABG.[13, 14] These investigators have also demonstrated a variety of changes in atrial refractoriness and conduction latency in patients undergoing CABG that may predispose them to have atrial fibrillation develop.[14, 15] Sato et al. found prolongation of atrial conduction times during the first 2 hours after bypass in the canine heart.[16] Several groups have used prolonged P wave duration measured directly from the surface ECG or with signal averaging techniques as an index of intraatrial conduction delay and shown that it correlated with an increased incidence of postoperative atrial fibrillation.[17, 18] A practical limitation to relying on these observations for screening patients preoperatively is the lack of standardization of P-wave measurements and the absence of commercially available P-wave signal averaging equipment.

In patients undergoing CABG, a significant increase in epinephrine and norepinephrine levels may be measured for up to 3 days in the postoperative period.[19, 20] This hyperadrenergic state may contribute to increased automaticity and increased frequency of premature atrial contractions, serving as a "trigger" for episodes of atrial fibrillation. Postoperative withdrawal of β-adrenergic blockers has also been postulated as a predisposing cause. However, investigators have not been able to demonstrate any direct correlation between the elevation of catecholamines and the development of atrial fibrillation in patients.

The time course of the development of atrial fibrillation parallels the development of postoperative pericarditis, which through acute inflammation may alter atrial coupling and lead to transient structural or electrophysiologic changes that predispose patients to atrial fibrillation. It has been difficult to study the relationship between pericarditis and atrial fibrillation because the diagnosis of atrial pericarditis is dependent on relatively nonspecific clinical and ECG findings. The ability of pericarditis to induce atrial flutter and atrial fibrillation is clear from animal models. The sterile pericarditis model in dogs is a well-established animal model of atrial flutter that, as the name suggests, relies on pericardial inflammation from pericardiectomy and pericardial irritation to induce atrial flutter.[21] The high incidence of pericardial effusions (up to 85% in some studies), as well as the time course of pericarditis in animal models and humans, suggests that further investigation into the role of pericardial inflammation contributing to postoperative atrial fibrillation is necessary.[22, 23]

PREDICTORS OF POSTOPERATIVE ATRIAL FIBRILLATION

Multiple studies have shown an increased incidence of postoperative atrial fibrillation with advanced age.[24–26] This is consistent with epidemiologic studies that also show an increased incidence of atrial fibrillation with advancing age in the nonpostoperative setting.[27] The effect of age on the incidence of atrial fibrillation is striking and is consistently the most powerful predictor of postoperative atrial fibrillation. For example, in a review of more than 5,000 CABG patients, atrial fibrillation developed in only 3.7% of patients younger than 40 years, compared with 28% of patients 70 years or older (Fig 2). Two recent studies have confirmed these observations.[8, 9]

Other clinical risk factors predicting the development of atrial fibrillation include a history of congestive heart failure, a history of preoperative atrial fibrillation, and a history of chronic obstructive pulmonary disease.[25, 26, 28] Other variables, including preoperative

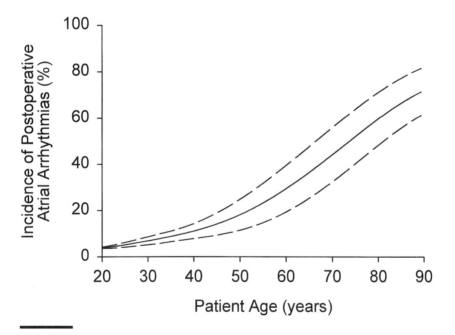

FIGURE 2.

Relationship between age and the incidence of atrial fibrillation. *Dashed lines* represent confidence intervals. (Courtesy of Creswell LL, Schuessler RB, Rosenbloom M, et al: Hazards of postoperative atrial arrhythmias. *Ann Thorac Surg* 56:539–549, 1993. Reprinted with permission from the Society of Thoracic Surgeons.)

use of β-blockers and digoxin, have not consistently been shown to signify decreased risk of developing atrial fibrillation.[28, 29]

Insight into the role of atrial preservation or atrial ischemia may be gained by searching for a relationship between the various aspects of surgical technique and their relationship to the incidence of atrial fibrillation.[30] One hypothesis proposes that atrial ischemia secondary to inadequate protection of atrial myocardium, or prolonged aortic cross clamp time may predispose patients to the development of postoperative atrial fibrillation. Several studies have shown an increased incidence of atrial fibrillation with increased cross-clamp or total pump time, but other studies have found no relationship.[9, 30] Other factors that may influence the incidence of atrial fibrillation are the type and volume of cardioplegia used to afford myocardial protection and the method of cannulation. Several small studies have examined the incidence of atrial fibrillation with cold cardioplegia, crystalloid cardioplegia, blood cardioplegia, intermittent aortic cross-clamping time, and diltiazem-containing cardioplegia.[31–33] No consistent or only small differences in the incidence of atrial fibrillation with different types of cardioplegia were discovered in these studies.

Considerable work is ongoing to further study the electrophysiologic effects of different methods of providing cardioplegia to the heart. The method of cardiac cannulation for delivery of cardioplegia will also affect atrial preservation. No clear-cut advantage has been demonstrated for single vs. bicaval cannulation on the incidence of atrial fibrillation.[9, 34]

Other surgical variables that have been associated with a higher incidence of atrial fibrillation include bypass grafting to the right coronary artery, concomitant right coronary artery endarterectomy, use of the internal mammary artery graft, pulmonary vein venting, and postoperative atrial pacing.[8, 9, 29] In a preliminary report from a large multicenter study, frequent preoperative premature atrial contractions (PACs) were a risk factor for post-CABG atrial fibrillation.[35] The major limitation to most of these studies is the small sample size or failure to determine whether the surgical variable is independent of poor left ventricular function and age. These issues will only be clarified by analyzing the results of large, prospective multicenter registries comparing different surgical techniques in patients at high risk for having postoperative atrial fibrillation develop.

The role of *preoperative* digoxin in changing the incidence of atrial fibrillation has been reviewed in several large series. In one large recent report of 2,833 patients undergoing CABG, the incidence of postoperative atrial fibrillation was 32% in patients not taking digoxin preoperatively and 44% in patients taking preoperative digoxin ($P < 0.001$).[24] In another study, preoperative use of digoxin was a univariate but not a multivariate predictor of the development of atrial fibrillation. The major limitation of these analyses is that the reason for preoperative digoxin use is often unclear. It is possible that most of these patients were taking digoxin because of a history of previous atrial fibrillation, which is also a risk factor for postoperative atrial fibrillation.

MEDICAL MANAGEMENT

Atrial fibrillation is easily diagnosed on the basis of rhythm strips or a 12-lead ECG. In some cases, it can only be differentiated from a variety of other supraventricular arrhythmias, including atypical atrial flutter, by recording intra-atrial electrograms from temporary atrial epicardial wires. In this situation, atrial fibrillation is characterized by the irregularity of intervals between atrial electrograms, and the variability in electrogram amplitude and morphology.

A general approach to the management of atrial fibrillation is outlined below. Most physicians will initiate treatment of patients with post-CABG atrial fibrillation lasting 15–30 minutes or associated with severe symptoms. Immediate or urgent therapy for atrial fibrillation consists of direct current (DC) cardioversion beginning with 200 J of synchronized (to the R wave) energy while the patient is sedated with midazolam or brevital. Urgent therapy is indicated for patients with hemodynamic instability who have hypotension, pulmonary edema, or severe unstable angina. Optimal results are obtained with self-adhesive patches to lower transthoracic impedance. A variety of chest placements have been used, with standard placements being cardiac apex-anterior, apex-posterior, and anterior-posterior.[36] These positions have been shown to be equally effective. Electrodes should not be placed on the breast in women, but rather lateral or below the breast. Atrial overdrive pacing can be instituted if atrial flutter is present. In the absence of the need to perform urgent cardioversion, strategies for the medical management of the post-CABG patient with atrial fibrillation include drugs to control the ventricular response, drugs to restore sinus rhythm and prevent recurrences of atrial fibrillation, and anticoagulation (Fig 3).

HEART RATE CONTROL

Atrial fibrillation with a rapid ventricular rate may cause chest pain, shortness of breath, dizziness, or other symptoms. A rapid

Post OP AF Treatment Algorithm

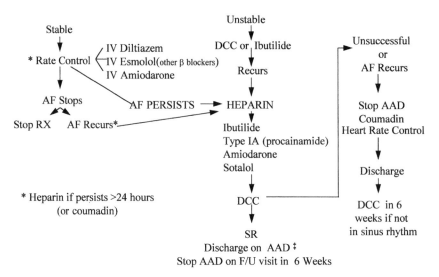

FIGURE 3.
Algorithm for management of postoperative patients with atrial fibrillation. *Abbreviations: AF,* atrial fibrillation; *Rx,* treatment; *DCC,* direct current cardioversion; *SR,* sinus rhythm.

ventricular response leads to a worsening of diastolic dysfunction because of a shortening of the diastolic filling period, loss of atrioventricular (AV) synchrony, decreased coronary perfusion time, as well as decreased cardiac output and elevated pulmonary wedge pressure. Heart rate control will improve hemodynamics in these patients if it is not associated with an excessive decrease in blood pressure. There are no comparative studies of the major agents (e.g., digoxin, β-blockers, calcium channel blockers) used for heart rate control in the post-CABG patient. Only limited experience is available with the use of clonidine or IV magnesium for heart rate control. In general, most acute therapy involves the use of IV calcium channel blockers (especially diltiazem) or IV β-blockers (e.g., esmolol) if hemodynamic tolerance permits for acute heart rate control. We recommend a target heart rate while resting supine of 60–100 beats/min (Table 1).

Digoxin is typically ineffective in this situation because of the high sympathetic tone characteristic of the postoperative pe-

TABLE 1.
Drugs Used for Heart Rate Control

Acute Rate Control	Drug	Dosing	Efficacy	Side Effects
Rapid heart rate; BP < 90 mm Hg	None	Immediate	Direct current cardioversion	Atrial fibrillation may recur
Rapid heart rate; Symptomatic	Diltiazem	IV bolus: 20 mg over 2 min; 25 mg IV over 2 min (if needed), then infuse 5–15 mg/hr	Prompt and very good heart rate control	Hypotension
	Verapamil	IV 5–10 mg, repeat after 10–15 min	Good heart rate control	Hypotension, negative inotrope, swings in heart rate control without maintenance infusion
	Esmolol	IV 0.5 mg/kg over 1 min, then infuse 0.05 mg/kg/min; may titrate up	Short acting, good heart rate control	Hypotension, asthma, exacerbation of heart failure
	Metoprolol (or Inderal)	IV 5 mg q 5 min; total 15 mg	Rapid rate control	Hypotension
	Digoxin	IV 0.25–0.5 mg (total: 1 mg/24 hr)	Moderate-to-low efficacy in this patient population	Delayed onset, toxicity
	Amiodarone	IV 150 mg/10 min, 1 mg/min × 6 hrs, then 0.5 mg/min	Prompt, works in patients on pressor or critically ill	Rare, occasionally mild hypotension with bolus

riod.[37, 38] In addition, the drug's relatively narrow toxic-therapeutic window predisposes to developing digoxin toxicity, especially when advanced age or renal impairment is present. When administered, up to 1 mg of IV digoxin can be given in the first 24 hours. Heart rate slowing effects are generally not seen for several hours. Intravenous β-blockade is effective for achieving rate control in many postoperative patients. Esmolol is often given in this situation because it has a short half-life and, thus, a rapid onset/offset of action. The main limitation to IV β-blockade is the relatively high incidence of hypotension (10% to 67%), especially in the postoperative setting.[39] In some centers, IV esmolol infusions or boluses of inderal or metoprolol are used for heart rate control. Intravenous inderal and metoprolol are both relatively inexpensive, and there is considerable experience with these agents also in the postoperative periods. The efficacy of a bolus of IV esmolol for heart rate control has been reported to be as high as 72%, but only 59% to 67% of patients have sustained heart rate control after 4 hours. In these trials, sinus rhythm was restored in only 14% to 16% of patients.

Intravenous calcium channel blockers have been used widely in the postoperative setting, with the major limiting factor also being hypotension (incidence 5% to 20%). We have had extensive experience with IV diltiazem in the postoperative setting.[40, 41] Intravenous diltiazem infusions can be easily titrated (5–15 mg/hr), infused safely for days to weeks, and provide prompt and sustained heart rate control in approximately 70% to 80% of patients. In our experience, heart rate control is generally achieved within 5–10 minutes after the bolus (20 mg over 2–3 minutes) is infused. A second bolus (25 mg) can be administered 15 minutes later if the first bolus provides inadequate heart rate control. We generally initiate a continuous maintenance infusion immediately after the bolus injection at 10 mg/hr and then titrate the infusion to 15 mg/hr, as needed. Higher doses have been rarely given (up to 20 mg/hr), but the incidence of hypotension may increase at this dose. Intravenous diltiazem can be safely and easily switched to the long-acting preparation.[42] Patients whose heart rates are controlled with 5 mg/hr can be switched to Cardiazem CD, 180 or 240 mg/day; patients receiving a 10 mg/hr infusion can be switched to 240–300 mg/day; and patients receiving 15 mg/hr for heart rate control may be switched to 300–360 mg/day. It is recommended that the first dose of sustained release diltiazem be given 6–8 hours before termination of the infusion. Diltiazem can generally be used safely in patients with mild or moderate heart failure, and IV or oral digoxin can be safely combined with diltiazem. Verapamil may also be infused intravenously; however, it has a greater negative inotropic and vasodilatory effect and increases digoxin levels.

Intravenous amiodarone may provide heart rate control and hemodynamic improvement in patients refractory to all other efforts at heart rate control. We have recently reported our experience with IV amiodarone in 38 critically ill patients refractory to conventional therapy for either heart rate control or to restore sinus rhythm.[43] These patients all had failed treatment with digoxin, β-blockers, calcium channel blockers, and procainamide alone or in combination. Intravenous amiodarone was administered as a 150-mg bolus over 10 minutes, followed by a 1 mg/min infusion for 6 hours, and then a 0.5 mg/min infusion for days to weeks. Before initiation of IV amiodarone, 20 patients had systolic hypotension (systolic blood pressure less than 100 mm Hg) and many were either receiving IV inotropes, vasopressors, or mechanical hemodynamic support before the onset of rapid atrial fibrillation. One third of this patient group had atrial fibrillation after CABG or a valve replacement. Heart rate control was achieved within 1 hour in the patients receiving IV amiodarone, without a decrease in blood pressure. In a subgroup of patients with invasive hemodynamic monitoring, the cardiac index increased by 12% and the pulmonary artery wedge pressure decreased from 22 ± 3 mm Hg to 20 ± 2 mm Hg after 1 hour of IV amiodarome. Our patients received IV amiodarone for 84 ± 79 hours, and all achieved satisfactory acute heart rate control. Based on our experience with this group of patients, we routinely use IV amiodarone for control of the heart rate in acute atrial fibrillation or atrial flutter in patients refractory or intolerant to conventional therapy.

RESTORATION AND MAINTENANCE OF SINUS RHYTHM

This is an important area for which there are many ongoing new trials. Direct current cardioversion is usually avoided in the postoperative setting because most episodes tend to be short and recurrent, thereby making it necessary to perform this procedure repeatedly. In addition, some surgeons express concern about the effect of cardioversion on sternal wound healing and postoperative pain. In some centers, however, DC cardioversion is performed fairly early, and antiarrhythmic drug therapy is saved for patients who have recurrences. In many centers, the mainstay of therapy consists of antiarrhythmic agents usually administered immediately before or after DC cardioversion. Nevertheless, DC cardioversion should be performed when necessary to urgently restore sinus rhythm as mentioned earlier.

A variety of antiarrhythmic agents have been shown to be more effective than placebo or digoxin in restoring sinus rhythm. In general, the percentage of patients reverting to sinus rhythm is high in both the group receiving antiarrhythmic agents and the group receiving placebo because the spontaneous reversion rate is high in this setting. For example, Hjelms compared IV procainamide to digoxin in 30 patients after CABG.[44] After 40 minutes, 87% of patients receiving procainamide and 60% of patients receiving placebo converted to sinus rhythm. Intravenous quinidine, propafenone, amiodarone, and sotalol have all been shown to be effective for restoration of sinus rhythm.[45–48] In one study, IV amiodarone was shown to be effective for restoring and maintaining sinus rhythm (often after DC cardioversion), as well as providing heart rate control in a group of 38 patients refractory to conventional therapy, whereas in other studies its efficacy is low.[43] The precise role of IV amiodarone in restoring sinus rhythm will await the results of several large, ongoing prospective studies in this patient population. It is our impression, however, that IV amiodarone has a relatively low efficacy for acute conversion to sinus rhythm but appears to be effective for maintaining sinus rhythm once patients are electrically cardioverted. In several studies, IV sotalol has been demonstrated to be effective for the restoration of sinus rhythm. In one study it was demonstrated to be equally efficacious to IV disopyramide, and in another study it was shown to be superior to IV metoprolol.[47, 48]

Intravenous ibutilide, a recently approved class-III agent with a short time to onset of action, has been shown to be effective for the acute termination of atrial fibrillation and atrial flutter.[49, 50] In comparative studies of largely nonpostoperative patients, ibutilide is more effective than IV procainamide or IV sotalol for termination of atrial flutter and atrial fibrillation.[49] The drug is administered as a 1-mg dose over 10 minutes, and can be repeated in 10 minutes if excessive QT prolongation has not occurred and the atrial arrhythmia has not terminated. For patients weighing less than 60 kg, the initial and subsequent infusion dose is 0.01 mg/kg. In controlled clinical trials, approximately 40% to 60% of patients with atrial fibrillation or flutter revert to sinus rhythm, with reversion occurring within 60 minutes in approximately 90% of patients. Its electrophysiologic effects last up to 4 hours. This agent is unusual because of its relatively high efficacy for restoration of sinus rhythm without associated hypotension. Based on our experience with this agent, we generally recommend IV ibutilide be administered to patients with postoperative atrial fibrillation that does not spontaneously resolve. Patients are given this agent only after the serum levels of potassium and magnesium are normal, and the QT interval corrected for heart rate (QT_c) is less than 450 msec. Additionally, patients with a history of torsade de pointes with other antiarrhythmic agents should not be given ibutilide. Continuous ECG monitoring for at least 4 hours after termination of the infusion or until the QT_c has returned to normal is recommended. We believe ibutilide is an ideal agent for this population because of its rapid onset, favorable hemodynamic profile, and high success rate. Its main drawback is the possibility of recurrent atrial fibrillation necessitating additional doses of ibutilide or short-term therapy with oral antiarrhythmics. Trials in this post-CABG patient population have been recently completed.

PROPHYLAXIS

A variety of agents have shown to be effective in preventing the occurrence of atrial fibrillation in this setting. The most solid evidence for atrial fibrillation prophylaxis exists for the effectiveness of β-blockers. In 1988, Lauer reported from a survey of chiefs of cardiothoracic surgery that 44% were using β-blockers for atrial fibrillation prophylaxis in the postoperative setting.[1] Hesitancy to use β-blockers probably represents the increasing prevalence of elderly patients with poor left ventricular function and other relative contraindications to β-blocker use among those who are now currently undergoing CABG.

A variety of β-blockers including propanolol, timolol, metoprolol, nadolol, and acebutolol have been found effective when administered postoperatively to prevent or decrease the number of episodes of atrial fibrillation.[51–53] Two meta-analyses of β-blockers have confirmed the beneficial effects of their prophylactic administration. Andrews et al. selected 24 of 69 studies that had adequate control groups or proper randomization procedures and reported a decrease in the incidence of post-CABG atrial fibrillation from 34% to 8.7% ($P < 0.0001$) in 1,549 patients receiving prophylactic β-blockers.[54] Their analysis suggested β-blocker therapy was of most benefit in patients at greatest risk of hemodynamic compromise from atrial fibrillation (e.g., those patients with left ventricular dysfunction). Kowey's meta-analysis of 7 trials included 2,482 patients and showed a reduction in the incidence of supraventricular arrhythmias from 20% to 9.8% in patients taking β-blockers ($P < 0.001$).[55] Various definitions of atrial fibrillation are used in different studies, with some varying from 30 seconds to several minutes in length. The effect of the time of initiation and dose of β-blocker on the incidence of atrial fibrillation does not seem to be important. A final concern we have is the relevance of applying the results of studies done mostly during 1970–1980 to the current practice of cardiac surgery. The patients now being operated on are older, sicker, and have more severe underlying cardiac disease. Additional trials are needed to determine the safety and efficacy of β-blocker prophylaxis in this patient population.

Digoxin does not appear to have a consistent effect on the prevention of *postoperative* atrial fibrillation.[56, 57] Meta-analyses of the prophylactic trials using digoxin showed no significant benefit of digoxin use in the prevention of atrial fibrillation. There are no placebo-controlled, double-blind trials of digoxin as a prophylactic agent for atrial fibrillation. A combination of digoxin and β-blockers caused a greater reduction in the incidence of atrial fibrillation, suggesting a possible synergism between the two agents.

Studies with oral verapamil and a meta-analysis of oral verapamil have failed to show any effect of this agent on preventing atrial fibrillation.[54, 58, 59] Oral verapamil was, however, shown to cause a lower ventricular rate, but higher rates of hypotension and pulmonary edema were also seen. In a small randomized study of IV diltiazem vs. IV nitroglycerin, there was a lower incidence of atrial fibrillation in the patients who received IV diltiazem.[60]

Studies of the efficacy of magnesium in preventing post-CABG atrial fibrillation have shown variable results. Two placebo-controlled trials of IV magnesium beginning immediately in the postoperative setting failed to show any benefit.[61, 62] Others have found a benefit of IV magnesium when levels were increased to 2.0 mEq/L or more, but in general this difference is small. The mechanisms by which magnesium may have an effect on the incidence of atrial fibrillation are unknown.

Intravenous procainamide was recently shown to be ineffective at reducing the incidence of atrial fibrillation, although it reduced the number of "atrial fibrillation days" patients spent in the hospital.[63] In contrast, sotalol has been shown to be effective in a number of studies in lowering the incidence of postoperative atrial fibrillation.[47, 64] Intravenous amiodarone has also been shown to be effective in a small, prospective, randomized, placebo-controlled study of 77 patients, lowering the incidence of atrial fibrillation from 21% to 5%.[65] A larger randomized trial of IV amiodarone is underway for prophylaxis of atrial fibrillation.

The role of atrial pacing in patients with sick sinus syndrome has been studied retrospectively in the nonpostoperative patient. It is believed that atrial pacing decreases the incidence of atrial fibrillation in patients with the sick sinus syndrome who have indications for permanent pacing. Recently, some data have suggested an additional protective effect of biatrial pacing compared with pacing the right atrium alone.[66] It is common clinical practice to perform overdrive atrial pacing in the postoperative period to suppress atrial ectopy and provide optimal hemodynamics. A recent preliminary report from a randomized, controlled clinical trial of atrial overdrive pacing (AAI pacing mode) at rates greater than or equal to 10 beats/min faster than the intrinsic heart rate (i.e., approximately 90–110 beats/min) did not prevent postoperative atrial fibrillation.[67] Future studies must address whether biatrial pacing has any benefit in the prevention of atrial fibrillation.

ANTICOAGULATION

The risk of a stroke in the setting of chronic atrial fibrillation is one of the most well-studied issues in clinical medicine. However, relatively little information about the risk of stroke in patients who have postoperative atrial fibrillation exists.

The general incidence of stroke has been reported to range from 1% to 3% in patients after CABG.[68, 69] Multiple studies have shown a clear association between postoperative atrial fibrillation and postoperative stroke or transient ischemic attack. In one study by Taylor et al., 453 consecutive patients undergoing CABG were followed up prospectively, and stroke or transient ischemic attack occurred in 10 patients (2.2%).[70] Only two factors predicted stroke in a multivariate analysis: a history of stroke or transient ischemic attack, and postoperative atrial fibrillation. Strokes occurred in 6 (7%) of 86 patients with postoperative atrial fibrillation compared with 4 (1%) of 367 patients without postoperative atrial fibrillation ($P < 0.005$). Similar findings were obtained by Reed et al. in patients who underwent CABG between 1970 and 1984.[71] These investigators found an odds ratio for the increased risk of stroke of 3.0 in patients with postoperative atrial fibrillation. Creswell et al. also showed that post-CABG atrial fibrillation was associated with an increased incidence of a postoperative stroke (3.3% vs. 1.4%, $P < 0.0005$).[25] Arnold and colleagues from the Cleveland Clinic retrospectively reviewed the records of patients undergoing DC cardioversion for atrial fibrillation lasting more than 48 hours.[72] Two of 115 postoperative patients not anticoagulated had a stroke, and 0 of 101 patients anticoagulated had a stroke.

Based on these studies, as well as transesophageal studies, it seems that the risk of embolic strokes is substantial after 48 hours or more of atrial fibrillation.[73] Patients with post-CABG atrial fibrillation should be anticoagulated unless a contraindication exists. The role of transesophageal echocardiography to minimize the risk of thromboembolic events in patients with contraindications to anticoagulation is being studied.

FINANCIAL IMPLICATIONS

Increased emphasis has been placed on the financial implications and resource utilization in patients with post-CABG atrial fibrillation. Several recent studies have highlighted the nature of increased costs associated with this postoperative complication. These increased costs have been primarily related to increased duration of hospitalization, increased duration of ICU hospitalization, increased laboratory costs, and increased pharmacy costs in some studies. The total increase in charges in one study was more than $8,000 or almost 16%.[74] Hospital stays are generally increased by a minimum of 2 or 3 days by postoperative atrial fibrillation. A recently published study attributed an additional 4.9 days of hospitalization to the occurrence of postoperative atrial fibrillation, with

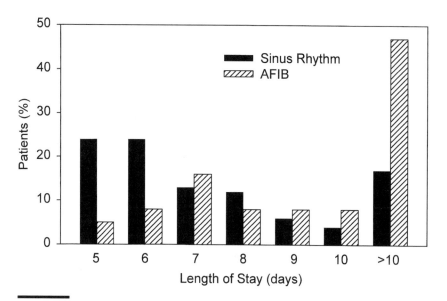

FIGURE 4.
Relationship between duration of hospitalization and development of postoperative atrial fibrillation *(AFIB)*. (Courtesy of Aranki SF, Shaw DP, Adams DH, et al: Predictors of atrial fibrillation after coronary artery surgery. Current trends and impact on hospital resources. *Circulation* 94:390–397. Copyright 1996, American Heart Association. Reproduced with permission.)

an increase in hospital charges of $10,000 or more (Fig 4).[8, 9] With increased pressures to perform CABG and accelerate recovery and discharge, the impact of atrial fibrillation on costs and lengths of stay is likely to remain an important concern.

CONCLUSION

Atrial fibrillation after CABG remains a major problem that is likely to increase, because the typical patient undergoing CABG is older and sicker than the typical patient was 10–20 years ago. With physicians and hospitals facing increasing pressure to control costs, the future of therapy for this condition lies in prophylaxis. Although β-blockers have been shown to be effective as single agents and in combination with digoxin, they are inconsistently used because of their many side effects and contraindications. Future improvements will result from identification and control of intraoperative factors to reduce the incidence of postoperative atrial fibrillation, as well as better prophylactic regimens that probably will still involve the use of antiarrhythmic drugs. Acute management will be focused on prompt reversion to sinus rhythm with acute infusions of agents such as ibutilide. Novel strategies such as postoperative atrial or biatrial pacing will need to be tested in this patient population. Potential agents such as nonsteroidal anti-inflammatory drugs designed to prevent pericarditis may also lower the incidence of postoperative atrial fibrillation.

REFERENCES

1. Lauer MS, Eagle KA, Buckley MJ, et al: Atrial fibrillation following coronary artery bypass surgery. *Prog Cardiovasc Dis* 16:367–378, 1989.
2. Asher C, Chung M, Eagle KA, et al: Atrial fibrillation following cardiac surgery, in Falk R, Podrid P (eds): *Atrial Fibrillation.* New York, Lippincott-Raven Press, in press.
3. Favaloro RG, Effler DB, Groves LK, et al: Direct myocardial revascularization with saphenous vein autograft. *Dis Chest* 56:279–283, 1969.
4. Goldman L: Supraventricular tachyarrhythmias in hospitalized adults after surgery. *Chest* 73:450–454, 1978.
5. Johnston KW: Multicenter prospective study of nonruptured abdominal aortic aneurysm. *J Vasc Surg* 9:437–447, 1989.
6. Nielsen JB, Sorensen HR, Alstrup P: Atrial fibrillation following thoracotomy for non-cardiac diseases, in particular cancer of the lung. *Acta Med Scand* 193:425–429, 1973.
7. Asher CR, Chung MK, Grimm RA, et al: Is the incidence of postoperative atrial fibrillation following cardiac valve surgery reduced by minimally invasive surgery (abstract). *Circulation* 94:651, 1996.

8. Aranki SF, Shaw DP, Adams DH, et al: Predictors of atrial fibrillation after coronary artery surgery: Current trends and impact on hospital resources. *Circulation* 94:390–397, 1996.

9. Matthew JP, Parks R, Savino JS, et al: Atrial fibrillation following coronary artery bypass graft surgery: Predictors, outcomes, and resource utilization. *JAMA* 276:300–306, 1996.

10. Fuller JA, Adams GG, Buxton B: Atrial fibrillation after coronary artery bypass grafting: Is it a disorder of the elderly? *J Thorac Cardiovasc Surg* 97:821–825, 1989.

11. Moe GK: On the multiple wavelet hypothesis of atrial fibrillation. *Arch Int Pharmacodyn Ther* 140:183–188, 1962.

12. Konings K, Kirchof CJJ, Smeets JRLM, et al: High density mapping of electrically induced atrial fibrillation in humans. *Circulation* 89:1665–1680, 1994.

13. Pool DP, Lee HL, Nadzam G, et al: Cardiac surgery results in changes of atrial refractoriness that may explain vulnerability to postoperative atrial fibrillation (abstract). *J Am Coll Cardiol* 27:64–65, 1995.

14. Chung MK, Pool DP, Leo HL, et al: Atrial conduction latency predicts occurrence of postoperative atrial fibrillation in patients undergoing bypass surgery (abstract). *J Am Coll Cardiol* 27:65A, 1995.

15. Augostini RS, Pool DP, Leo HL, et al: Sinus node function after cardiopulmonary bypass predicts the development of postoperative atrial fibrillation (abstract). *Circulation* 92:141, 1995.

16. Sato S, Yamauchi S, Schuessler RB, et al: The effect of augmented atrial hypothermia on atrial refractory period, conduction, and atrial flutter/fibrillation in the canine heart. *J Thorac Cardiovasc Surg* 104:297–306, 1992.

17. Buxton AE, Josephson ME: The role of P wave duration as a predictor of postoperative atrial arrhythmias. *Chest* 80:68–73, 1981.

18. Hutchinson LA, Ehlert FA, Menchavez-Tan E, et al: Towards a better understanding of the development of atrial fibrillation after cardiac surgery: Risk factor analysis in a large prospective study (abstract). *J Am Coll Cardiol* 27:318A, 1995.

19. Kyosola AU, Mattila K, Harjula T, et al: Life threatening complications of cardiac operations and occurrence of myocardial catecholamine bombs. *J Thorac Cardiovasc Surg* 95:334–339, 1988.

20. Engelman RM, Haag B, Lemeshow S, et al: Mechanism of plasma catecholamine increases during coronary artery bypass and valve procedures. *J Thorac Cardiovasc Surg* 86:608–615, 1983.

21. Page P, Plumb VJ, Okumura K, et al: A new model of atrial flutter. *J Am Coll Cardiol* 8:872–879, 1986.

22. Angelini GD, Penny WJ, El-Ghamary F, et al: The incidence and significance of early pericardial effusion after open heart surgery. *Eur J Cardiothorac Surg* 1:165–168, 1987.

23. Weitzman LB, Tinker WP, Kronzon I, et al: The incidence and natural history of pericardial effusion after cardiac surgery: An echocardiographic study. *Circulation* 69:506–511, 1984.

24. Leitch JW, Thomson D, Baird DK, et al: The importance of age as a predictor of atrial fibrillation and flutter after coronary artery bypass grafting. *J Thorac Cardiovasc Surg* 100:338–342, 1990.

25. Creswell LL, Schuessler RB, Rosenbloom M, et al: Hazards of postoperative atrial arrhythmias. *Ann Thorac Surg* 56:539–549, 1993.

26. Frost L, Molgaard H, Christiansen EH, et al: Atrial fibrillation and flutter after coronary artery bypass surgery: Epidemiology, risk factors and preventive trials. *Int J Cardiol* 36:253–261, 1992.

27. Kannel WB, Abbott RD, Savage DD, et al: Epidemiologic features of chronic atrial fibrillation: The Framingham Study. *N Engl J Med* 206:1018–1022, 1982.

28. Crosby LH, Pifalo WB, Woll KR, et al: Risk factors for atrial fibrillation after coronary artery bypass grafting. *Am J Cardiol* 66:1520–1522, 1990.

29. Omerod OM, McGregor CA, Stone DL, et al: Arrhythmias after coronary bypass surgery. *Br Heart J* 51:618–621, 1984.

30. Dixon FE, Genton E, Vacek JL, et al: Factors predisposing to supraventricular tachyarrhythmias after coronary artery bypass grafting. *Am J Cardiol* 58:476–478, 1986.

31. Butler J, Chong JL, Rocker GM, et al: Atrial fibrillation after coronary artery bypass grafting: A comparison of cardioplegia versus intermittent aortic cross-clamping. *Eur J Cardiothorac Surg* 7:23–25, 1983.

32. Pattison C, Dimitri WR, Williams BT: Dysrhythmias following coronary artery surgery: A comparison between cold cardioplegic and intermittent ischaemic arrest (32 C) with the effect of right coronary artery endarterectomy. *J Cardiovasc Surg* 29:601–605, 1988.

33. Muller JC, Khan N, Weisel RD, et al: Atrial activity during cardioplegia and postoperative arrhythmias. *J Thorac Cardiovasc Surg* 94:558–565, 1987.

34. Cheung EH, Arcidi JM, Jackson ER, et al: Intracavitary right heart cooling during coronary bypass surgery, a prospective randomized trial. *Circulation* 78:173S–179S, 1988.

35. Bigger JT Jr, Bloomfield DM, Rottman JN, et al: Frequent pre-operative atrial premature complexes predicts atrial fibrillation after CABG surgery (abstract). *Circulation* 94:191, 1996.

36. Pagan-Carlo LA, Spencer KT, Roberson CE, et al: Transthoracic defibrillation: Importance of avoiding electrode placement directly on the female breast. *J Am Coll Cardiol* 27:449–452, 1996.

37. Gilligan DM, Ellenbogen KA, Epstein AE: The management of atrial fibrillation. *Am J Med* 101:413–421, 1996.

38. Galun E, Flugelman MY, Glickson M, et al: Failure of long-term digitalization to prevent rapid ventricular response in patients with paroxysmal atrial fibrillation. *Chest* 99:1038–1040, 1991.

39. Schwartz M, Michelson EL, Sawin HS, et al: Esmolol: Safety and efficacy in postoperative cardiothoracic patients with supraventricular tachyarrhythmias. *Chest* 93:705–711, 1988.

40. Ellenbogen KA, Dias VC, Plumb VJ, et al: A placebo-controlled trial of continuous intravenous diltiazem infusion for 24 hour heart rate control during atrial fibrillation and atrial flutter: A multicenter study. *J Am Coll Cardiol* 18:891–897, 1991.

41. Ellenbogen KA, Dias VC, Cardello FP, et al: Safety and efficacy of intravenous diltiazem in atrial fibrillation or atrial flutter. *Am J Cardiol* 75:45–49, 1995.

42. Blackshear JL, Stambler BS, Strauss WE, et al: Control of heart rate during transition from intravenous to oral diltiazem in atrial fibrillation or flutter. *Am J Cardiol* 78:1246–1250, 1996.

43. Clemo HF, Wood MA, Shepard RK, et al: Intravenous amiodarone for heart rate control in unstable atrial tachyarrhythmias (abstract). *Circulation* 94:665–666, 1996.

44. Hjelms E: Procainamide conversion of acute atrial fibrillation after open-heart surgery compared with digoxin treatment. *Scand J Thorac Cardiovasc Surg* 26:193–196, 1992.

45. McAlister HF, Luke RA, Whitlock RM, et al: Intravenous amiodarone bolus versus oral quinidine for atrial flutter and fibrillation after cardiac operations. *J Thorac Cardiovasc Surg* 99:911–918, 1990.

46. Gentili C, Giordano F, Alois A, et al: Efficacy of intravenous propafenone in acute trial fibrillation complicating open-heart surgery. *Am Heart J* 123:1225–1228, 1992.

47. Suttorp MJ, Kingma JK, Peels HO, et al: Effectiveness of sotalol in preventing supraventricular tachyarrhythmias shortly after coronary artery bypass grafting. *Am J Cardiol* 68:1163–1169, 1991.

48. Campbell TJ, Gavaghan TP, Morgan JJ: Intravenous sotalol for the treatment of atrial fibrillation and atrial flutter after cardiopulmonary bypass: Comparison with disopyramide and digoxin in a randomized trial. *Br Heart J* 54:86–90, 1985.

49. Ellenbogen KA, Stambler BS, Wood MA, et al: Efficacy of intravenous ibutilide for rapid termination of atrial fibrillation and atrial flutter: A dose-response study. *J Am Coll Cardiol* 28:130–136, 1996.

50. Ellenbogen KA, Clemo HF, Stambler BS, et al: Efficacy of ibutilide for termination of atrial fibrillation and flutter. *Am J Cardiol* 78:42S–45S, 1996.

51. Matangi MF, Neutze JM, Grahm KJ, et al: Arrhythmia prophylaxis after aorta-coronary bypass: The effect of minidose propranolol. *J Thorac Cardiovasc Surg* 89:439–443, 1985.

52. Martinussen HJ, Lolk A, Szczepanski C, et al: Supraventricular tachyarrhythmias after coronary bypass surgery: A double blind randomized trial of prophylactic low dose propranolol. *Thorac Cardiovasc Surg* 36:206–207, 1988.

53. Khuri SF, Okike ON, Josa M, et al: Efficacy of nadolol in preventing supraventricular tachycardia after coronary artery bypass grafting. *Am J Cardiol* 60:51D–58D, 1987.

54. Andrews TC, Reimold SC, Berlin JA, et al: Prevention of supraventricular arrhythmias after coronary artery bypass surgery: A meta-analysis of randomized control trials. *Circulation* 84:236S–244S, 1991.

55. Kowey PR, Taylor JE, Rials SJ, et al: Meta-analysis of the effectiveness of prophylactic drug therapy in preventing supraventricular arrhythmia early after coronary artery bypass grafting. *Am J Cardiol* 69:863–865, 1992.

56. Johnson LW, Dickstein RA, Fruehan CT, et al: Prophylactic digitalization for coronary artery bypass surgery. *Circulation* 53:819–822, 1976.

57. Tyras DH, Stothert JC, Kaiser GC, et al: Supraventricular tachyarrhythmias after myocardial revascualrization: A randomized trial of prophylactic digitalization. *J Thorac Cardiovasc Surg* 77:310–313, 1979.

58. Davison R, Hartz R, Kaplan K, et al: Prophylaxis of supraventricular tachyarrhythmia after coronary bypass surgery with oral verapamil: A randomized double-blind trial. *Ann Thorac Surg* 39:336–339, 1985.

59. Smith EJ, Shore DF, Monro JL, et al: Oral verapamil fails to prevent supraventricular tachycardia following coronary artery surgery. *Int J Cardiol* 9:37–44, 1985.

60. Seitelberger R, Hannes W, Gleichauf M, et al: Effects of diltiazem on perioperative ischemia, arrhythmias, and myocardial function in patients undergoing elective coronary bypass grafting. *J Thorac Cardiovasc Surg* 107:811–821, 1994.

61. Fanning WJ, Thomas CS, Roach A, et al: Prophylaxis of atrial fibrillation with magnesium sulfate after coronary artery bypass grafting. *Ann Thorac Surg* 52:529–533, 1991.

62. Parikka H, Toivonen L, Pellinen T, et al: The influence of intravenous magnesium sulphate on the occurrence of atrial fibrillation after coronary artery bypass operation. *Eur Heart J* 14:251–258, 1993.

63. Gold MR, O'Gara PT, Buckley MJ, et al: Efficacy and safety of procainamide in preventing arrhythmias after coronary artery bypass surgery. *Am J Cardiol* 78:975–979, 1996.

64. Nystrom U, Edvardsson N, Berggren H, et al: Oral sotalol reduces the incidence of atrial fibrillation after coronary artery bypass graft surgery. *J Thorac Cardiovasc Surg* 41:34–37, 1993.

65. Hohnloser SH, Meinertz T, Dammbacher T, et al: Electrocardiographic and antiarrhythmic effects of intravenous amiodarone: Results of a prospective, placebo-controlled study. *Am Heart J* 121:89–95, 1991.

66. Saksena S, Prakash A, Hill M, et al: Prevention of recurrent atrial fibrillation with chronic dual-site right atrial pacing. *J Am Coll Cardiol* 28:687–694, 1996.

67. Chung MK, Augostini RS, Asher CR, et al: A randomized controlled study of atrial overdrive pacing for the prevention of atrial fibrillation after coronary bypass surgery (abstract). *Circulation* 69:188, 1996.

68. Loop FD, Cosgrove DM, Lytle BW, et al: An 11 year evolution of coronary arterial surgery (1968–1978). *Ann Surg* 190:444–455, 1979.

69. Gardner TJ, Horneffer PJ, Manolio TA, et al: Stroke following coronary artery bypass grafting: A ten year study. *Ann Thorac Surg* 40:574–581, 1985.

70. Taylor GJ, Malik SA, Colliver JA, t al: Usefulness of atrial fibrillation as a predictor of stroke after isolated coronary artery bypass grafting. *Am J Cardiol* 60:905–907, 1987.

71. Reed GL, Singer DE, Picard EH, et al: Stroke following coronary artery bypass surgery. *N Engl J Med* 319:1246–1250, 1988.
72. Arnold AZ, Mick MJ, Mazurek RP, et al: Role of prophylactic anticoagulation for direct current cardioversion in patients with atrial fibrillation and atrial flutter. *J Am Coll Cardiol* 13:617–623, 1989.
73. Manning WJ, Leeman DE, Gotch PJ, et al: Pulsed Doppler evaluation of atrial mechanical function after electrical conversion of atrial fibrillation. *J Am Coll Cardiol* 13:617–623, 1989.
74. Mauldin PD, Weintraub WS, Becker ER: Predicting hospital costs for first time coronary artery bypass grafting from preoperative and postoperative variables. *Am J Cardiol* 74:772–775, 1994.

CHAPTER 8

Left Ventricular Assist

O.H. Frazier, M.D.
Co-Director, Cullen Cardiovascular Research Laboratories, Texas Heart
Institute; Chief, Cardiopulmonary Transplantation, Texas Heart Institute
and St. Luke's Episcopal Hospital; Professor, Department of Surgery, The
University of Texas—Houston Medical School, Houston, Texas

T he field of mechanical circulatory support has never been
more promising. Each year, more lives are saved by short- and
long-term assist devices. Many of the problems with this technology that plagued researchers in the 1960s have been resolved. Others are close to being conquered. All told, cardiac assistance has
become a viable means of treating patients with ailing hearts.

Currently, a variety of mechanical assist devices are available
for use in patients who need ventricular support. Selection among
these devices often depends on the length of the support needed.
Devices such as the ABIOMED BVS 5000 (ABIOMED Cardiovascular, Inc., Danvers, Mass), the Biomedicus (Bio-Medicus, Eden
Prairie, Minn), and the Hemopump (DIP, Medtronic, Grand Rap-
ids, Mich) are generally used for short-term support in patients
with acute heart failure. The Thoratec (Thoratec Corp., Berkeley,
Calif), Novacor (Baxter Healthcare Corp., Novacor Division, Oak-
land, Calif), and HeartMate (Thermo Cardiosystems, Inc., Woburn,
Mass), on the other hand, may be used for long-term support in
patients with chronic heart failure.

SHORT-TERM DEVICES

DESCRIPTIONS

ABIOMED BVS 5000 Assist Device

The ABIOMED BVS 5000 is an external, pulsatile assist device that
can be used for short-term (up to 2 weeks) support of either one or
both of the heart's ventricles. The device is generally used to treat
patients with postcardiotomy ventricular dysfunction or with cardiogenic shock after acute myocardial infarction; however, it has
also been used as a bridge to transplantation.[1, 2]

The device is made up of three parts: the pneumatic drive console, the transthoracic cannulas, and the disposable external blood pumps. This simple design requires minimal supervision by the device operator, making it a good alternative for community hospitals that lack the resources to operate more complicated devices.

The pneumatic drive console contains a microprocessor that controls the system. The console is self-regulated, automatically adjusting the pump rate of flow and the systolic/diastolic ratio. One console can be used to control either one or two blood pumps. If two pumps are being used, the console controls the right and left pumps separately.

The wire-reinforced, transthoracic cannulas are inserted into the left atrium and ascending aorta for support of the left ventricle and/or into the right atrium and pulmonary artery for support of the right ventricle. Each cannula is covered with Dacron at the point where the cannula exits the chest wall. Gravity is used to drain blood from the atrium into the pump. Care must be taken to place the blood pumps at the correct height (usually 25 cm below the atria) or prolonged filling may occur.

Each disposable blood pump supports one ventricle and contains an atrial and a ventricular polyurethane (Angioflex, ABIOMED Cardiovascular, Inc., Danvers, Mass) bladder. To ensure unidirectional blood flow, trileaflet valves are placed between the atrial and ventricular bladders and between the ventricular bladder and outflow cannula. A drive line connects the pump to the console. This drive line transfers compressed air from the console to the blood pump, thus collapsing the bladders and pushing blood through the inflow cannula.

COMPLICATIONS.—Because the cannulas are exteriorized, one of the most common complications associated with the BVS 5000 is infection. Most of these infections, however, are superficial. Furthermore, because the cannulas are covered in Dacron, the skin may grow into the Dacron surface, forming fibrotic tissue and protecting against infection. An additional potential complication is bleeding, because the patients are given anticoagulants to guard against thromboembolism.

RESULTS.—Results with this device have been good. Thus far, more than 500 patients have received ventricular assistance from a BVS 5000. Of those patients, 53% were postcardiotomy patients and 65% required biventricular support. Only 27% of the postcardiotomy patients were discharged, whereas more than 40% of the cardiomyopathy patients were discharged.[3] In addition, a report by

Guyton et al.[4] determined that of patients who had not had a cardiac arrest, the survival rate was 47%. According to the BVS Worldwide Registry, as of August 1995, 157 patients had been supported with the ABIOMED BVS 5000 as a bridge to transplantation. Ninety-one (57%) of these patients were discharged from the hospital (personal communication, ABIOMED, Danvers, Mass, August 11, 1995).

Biomedicus Pump

The Biomedicus Pump is a short-term, centrifugal device. The pump is external and can be used for either univentricular or biventricular support. The pump consists of acrylic rotator cones that produce continuous flow. Pump speed is controlled by a driver that is attached magnetically to the pump.[5] Because only cannulas are implanted within the body, this device can be used to support children. In these small patients, a 48-mL BP-50 model of the pump is used, whereas in adults an 80-mL BP-80 is used, which provides up to 10 L of flow per minute.

The pump is generally used in the postcardiotomy patient if weaning from cardiopulmonary bypass cannot be achieved, and if the maximum pharmacologic support and intra-aortic support is not sufficient.[6, 7] However, the pump may also be used to bridge some patients to transplantation or to revive them from acute cardiogenic shock.

For left ventricular support, the cannula may be inserted through the right superior pulmonary vein. In this manner, blood flows to the aorta through the aortic cannulation site. For right ventricular support, the cannula may be inserted in the right atrial appendage, with blood returning either through the pulmonary artery or through the angle of the right ventricle. Both methods may be implemented at the same time for biventricular support.

In addition, the pump may be connected to the heart through the bifurcated graft technique. A bifurcated graft is attached to the aorta. A cannula is passed through each limb of the graft: one that decompresses the left ventricle through the aortic valve, and another that returns the blood to the heart.

The main disadvantage of this pump is that it was designed to be used for only 48 hours. Possible complications include infection (because of the exteriorized cannulas) and thromboembolism (because of electromagnetic flow probes and connectors). Anticoagulants are generally not given to postcardiotomy patients supported by the pump, because bleeding is the primary complication within this patient group. When the danger of bleeding has passed, however, anticoagulants should be administered along with heparin sodium to prevent thromboembolism.

At our institution, the survival rate of patients supported with the Biomedicus is approximately 25%. This survival rate is comparable to that of other studies: Noon[8] reported a survival rate of 21%, and Killen and colleagues[9] reported a survival rate of 19.5%.

Although the Biomedicus centrifugal pump has also been used successfully as a bridge to cardiac transplantation both by us (O.H. Frazier, unpublished data) and by others,[10] its use for this purpose is becoming less frequent.[11]

Hemopump

The Hemopump is a small, easily insertable axial flow device. The actual pump is about the size of a pencil eraser. Despite its small size, however, the hemopump is capable of pumping 4.7 L of blood per minute. To provide this flow, the pump rotates at a speed of 25,000 rpm. Initially there was concern that such speed might cause hemolysis; however, the Hemopump appears to cause only minimal hemolysis (about the same as a pulsatile pump).

Insertion of the Hemopump can be achieved without major surgery.[12] In some cases, insertion of the device takes less than a minute. The pump is mounted on a catheter and is usually inserted through the femoral or iliac artery. The inflow cannula is placed within the left ventricle, drawing blood out of the ventricle and propelling it into the aorta.[13] Because it is positioned within the ventricular cavity, the Hemopump can directly unload the ventricle.

At present, there are three models of the Hemopump available: the femoral Hemopump (24F), the sternotomy Hemopump (26F), and the percutaneous Hemopump (14F). Although the Hemopump can be used only according to research protocol in the United States, it is in clinical use in Europe.

The pilot study of the Hemopump was performed at the Texas Heart Institute (THI). Seven patients in cardiogenic shock had the Hemopump implanted. Infection, vascular injury, and thrombosis did not occur in any of the patients while they were being supported by the pump.[14]

The first patient who received a Hemopump at THI was having severe cardiac allograft rejection. After 2 days of Hemopump support and treatment with OKT3, we were able to reverse the rejection. As this case demonstrates, the Hemopump is uniquely suited for heart transplant patients. Unlike the technique for implanting many of the pulsatile devices, implanting the Hemopump does not require that part of the myocardium be removed. In addition, insertion of the device is relatively noninvasive, saving the patient from another traumatic surgery and decreasing the risk of infection in these immunosuppressed patients.

Extensive study of the device was undertaken at the University of Texas Medical School at Houston where Merhige et al.[15] studied the effects of Hemopump support in dogs. They found that the pump lowered intraventricular cavitary pressures, allowing the ventricle to rest. This resting of the ventricle may allow damaged myocardium to recover and ventricular function to improve.

With these encouraging results, a multi-institutional study[16] was undertaken to evaluate the safety and efficacy of using the Hemopump to treat patients in cardiogenic shock. Of 41 patients who were successfully implanted with the Hemopump, 31.7% survived to 30 days. Overall, the hemodynamic status of the patients improved, cardiac index increased, and pulmonary capillary wedge pressure decreased. No leg ischemia occurred, and the patients had only minimal hemolysis.

When the Hemopump was first used clinically, the drive cable fractured in a few patients, causing the cannula to be ejected from the heart. Since then, the strength of the cable has been improved. Other possible complications include thromboembolism originating from the intraventricular mural thrombus that can occur in patients with cardiogenic shock. To date, no device-related thromboembolisms have occurred.

The Hemopump is an extremely versatile device. It is small enough to be inserted without a major operation, yet powerful enough to support 80% of a patient's circulation. Because of the ease of insertion, the Hemopump can be inserted quickly in patients who need immediate support. Furthermore, it can be inserted safely in heart transplant patients who may not be able to withstand the trauma and risk of infection that a major operation might bring.

Because patients supported by the Hemopump must remain in bed, it is not suited for long-term support. This element limits its use as a bridge to transplantation, because many transplant candidates endure lengthy waiting times for a donor organ. Other patients may require a more powerful device, one that can assume 100% of the ventricle's function. In such patients, a long-term pulsatile device may be more appropriate.

LONG-TERM CIRCULATORY SUPPORT

In the past decade, long-term pulsatile devices such as the Thoratec ventricular assist system (VAS), Novacor left ventricular assist system (LVAS), and HeartMate LVAS have become accepted methods of bridging patients to transplantation. These devices provide total support of a patient's circulation. Initially, they were used only to bridge patients to transplantation. Recently, however, these systems have begun to fulfill their original purpose as long-term alternatives to transplantation.

DEVICES

Thoratec Ventricular Assist System

First used clinically in 1976, the Thoratec VAS[17–19] was recently approved for general clinical use by the United States Food and Drug Administration (FDA). This system is pneumatically powered and may be used for partial or total support, for univentricular or biventricular support, and for bridging to transplantation or postcardiotomy weaning. This device has a stroke volume of 65 mL and a maximum output of 7 L/min.

The pump consists of a rigid polycarbonate housing that contains a flexible, seam-free, segmented sac. To ensure unidirectional flow, Bjork-Shiley concavo-convex tilting disc valves are located within the inlet and outlet portions of the pump. Left ventricular support is generally provided with either left atrial or left ventricular cannulation.

The system can function in one of three modes: volume, fixed-rate, and external-synchronous mode. The volume mode is the most commonly used. In this mode, a Hall sensor is used to measure the filling of the pump, which determines the pumping rate. The fixed-rate mode is used whenever a pump rate of 80 beats/min cannot be achieved. In this mode, the operator sets the pumping rate. In the external-synchronous mode, the patient's R-wave signals the pump to empty. This mode is used to wean patients from support by setting the heart rate ratio between 1:1 and 1:3.

The major disadvantage of the Thoratec is the extracorporeal location of the pumps; thus, patients supported by this device are relatively immobile. This disadvantage, however, may also be the Thoratec's greatest asset: because the system is extracorporeal, the amount of space required for implantation within the body is not an issue. Consequently, the Thoratec may be used to support the circulation of children and small adults.

As of January 1993, 211 bridge-to-transplant patients had been supported by the Thoratec VAS.[17] One hundred fifty-five (73%) of these patients required biventricular support; 54 (26%) required only left ventricular support. The other 2 patients required right ventricular support after cardiac allograft failure. Of the 211 patients, 136 (64%) underwent transplantation and 113 (54%) were discharged from the hospital. Thus, the early survival rate after transplantation was 83%, a rate comparable to that of patients treated conventionally before undergoing transplantation.

Novacor Left Ventricular Assist System

The Novacor LVAS is an implantable, pulsatile device that is used to bridge patients to cardiac transplantation.[18, 20] The blood pump consists of a seamless polyurethane sac that is compressed by dual pusher plates. To maintain unidirectional flow, the inflow and outflow conduits each contain a 21-mm bioprosthetic valve. The pump can produce a stroke volume of up to 70 mL.

The drive console is attached to the pump with a 20-foot cable. The console monitors the system, displaying information it receives from transducers within the pump. Like the Thoratec, the Novacor operates in three different modes: the synchronized mode, the fill-to-empty mode, and the fixed-rate mode. In the synchronized mode, the pump diastole corresponds to the cardiac systole, thus providing maximal unloading of the ventricle. In the fill-to-empty mode, the pumping rate depends on the filling rate of the pump. This mode maximizes pump output. The last mode, the fixed-rate mode, is rarely used. In this mode, the operator sets the pumping rate.

Disadvantages of the Novacor include audibility of the device and limited patient mobility. However, a battery-powered, wearable version of the Novacor that significantly improves patient mobility is now available.[21]

In a recent study, 60% of 129 patients underwent successful transplantation after support with the Novacor. Of these patients, the 30-day survival rate was 82%, again comparable to that of transplant patients who did not receive an assist device.[22]

HeartMate Left Ventricular Assist System

The HeartMate LVAS (Thermo Cardiosystems, Inc., Woburn, Mass) is a long-term pulsatile blood pump used to support the ventricular function of patients with severe heart failure, especially those awaiting transplantation.[18, 20] The blood pump is made of a flexible polyurethane diaphragm enclosed within a rigid outer housing made of a titanium alloy (Fig 1). The blood-contacting surfaces of the pump are textured to promote the development of a pseudointimal lining. The development of such a lining reduces the risk of thromboembolic complications and hemolysis, reducing the need for antithrombolytic agents.

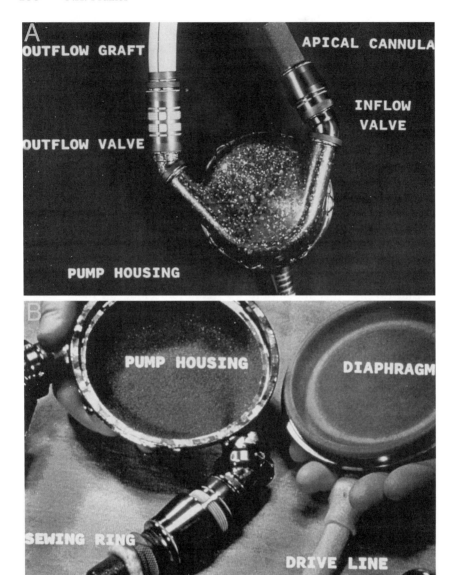

FIGURE 1.

A, the HeartMate implantable left ventricular assist system (LVAS). The apical cannula is placed within the left ventricle, the pump is placed in the left upper quadrant of the abdomen, and the outflow graft is anastomosed to the ascending aorta. **B,** the opened LVAS shows the textured titanium and polyurethane blood-contracting surfaces. (Courtesy of Myers TJ, Macris MP: Clinical experience with the HeartMate left ventricular assist device. *Heart Failure* 10:247–258, 1994. By permission of *Heart Failure*.)

The HeartMate comes in Implantable Pneumatic (IP) and Vented Electric (VE) models. Both systems incorporate the same blood pump and are placed in the same anatomical position (Fig 2). Both models have a maximum stroke volume of 85 mL. The IP-LVAS has a maximum blood flow of 12 L/min, whereas the VE-LVAS has a maximum blood flow of 10 L/min. The IP blood pump weighs 570 g and the VE blood pump weighs 1,150 g. The two models, however, differ mainly in their method of pump actuation (Fig 3). The IP-LVAS receives its power from an external drive console (Fig 4). The VE-LVAS receives its power from a lightweight, rechargeable battery pack through a percutaneous electric lead. The patient carries this battery pack on a shoulder holster, which allows greater mobility than the power console. Both models allow the patient to regain mobility while undergoing physical and hemodynamic rehabilitation, helping them become better candidates for heart transplantation.

The external drive console of the IP-LVAS is carried on a card and weighs 33 kg. A 6-foot cable connects the console to the pump. The pump can be used independent of the console for approximately 40 minutes at a time by using internal batteries. Recently, a new portable console powered by lead acid–gel batteries was introduced. It weighs 8.5 kg and can be transported with a shoulder strap or on wheels. Because this model is so portable, patients with these consoles may leave the hospital while supported with the HeartMate.

The VE-LVAS, on the other hand, is powered by an internal motor (Fig 5), which in turn is powered by either a stationary console or two lead-acid batteries. The motor is attached to either the console or the batteries by an electrical line, which in the new VE-LVAS shares a percutaneous lead with the vent tube.

Both the IP-LVAS and the VE-LVAS can be operated in the fixed-rate (rate set by the operator) or automatic (rate of flow adjusted to maintain an average stroke volume of approximately 75 mL) modes. The IP-LVAS also has a third mode: the external synchronous mode. In this mode, the patient's R-wave signals the pump to undergo systole.

PATIENT SELECTION

Patients who receive the Thoratec, Novacor, or HeartMate LVAS must fulfill similar criteria. To receive long-term mechanical circulatory support, patients must be in danger of dying or of end-organ failure. In addition, while the Thoratec may be used for both postcardiotomy weaning and bridging patients to transplantation,

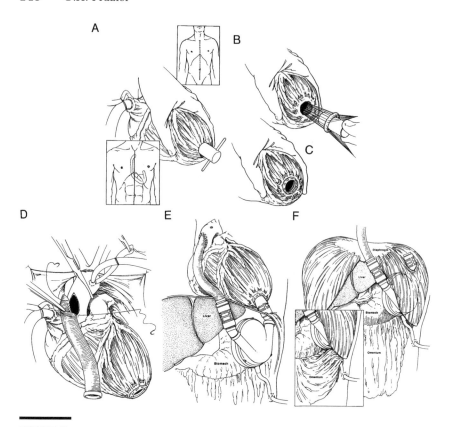

FIGURE 2.

Technique for implanting the HeartMate left ventricular assist system (LVAS). **A,** the left ventricular apex is cored with a circular knife. (*Insets* show median sternotomy with the extended abdominal incision and position of the pump. Note the position of the outlet graft in relation to the median sternotomy.) **B,** a Teflon-covered, reinforced Silastic sewing ring is secured to the apex with pledgeted sutures. **C,** sewing ring in place. **D,** the woven Dacron outlet graft is anastomosed end-to-side to the ascending aorta with a running 4-0 polypropylene suture. (Heart shown without pump in place.) **E,** the LVAS placed in the intra-abdominal, sub-diaphragmatic position. An opening in the diaphragm allows passage of the inlet tube from the pump to the left ventricle. The outlet graft lies above the diaphragm. **F,** position the pump (shown without connection to the heart) under the left diaphragmatic cupola. The *inset* shows omentum wrapped around the intra-abdominal portion of the drive line. (Courtesy of Radovancevic B, Frazier OH, Duncan MJ: Implantation technique for the HeartMate left ventricular assist device. *J Card Surg* 7:203–207, 1992. By permission of the *Journal of Cardiac Surgery.*)

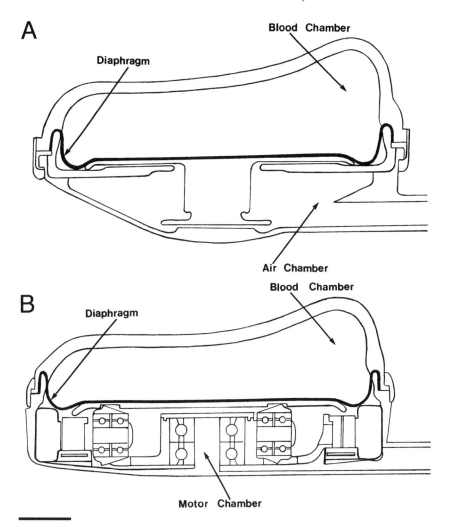

FIGURE 3.

Schematic drawings demonstrate the differences between the Implantable Pneumatic left ventricular assist system (IP-LVAS) and the Vented Electric LVAS
(VE-LVAS) pumps. The IP-LVAS **(A)** has an airspace located beneath the
diaphragm, and the VE-LVAS **(B)** has a low-speed torque motor. (Courtesy of Myers TJ, Macris MP: Clinical experience with the HeartMate left ventricular assist
device. *Heart Failure* 10:247–258, 1994. By permission of *Heart Failure.*)

the Novacor and the HeartMate are used only to bridge patients to
transplantation (or now as an alternative to transplantation).

Patients who receive long-term mechanical support generally
have heart failure that has not responded adequately to conventional inotropic drug and intra-aortic balloon pump treatment.

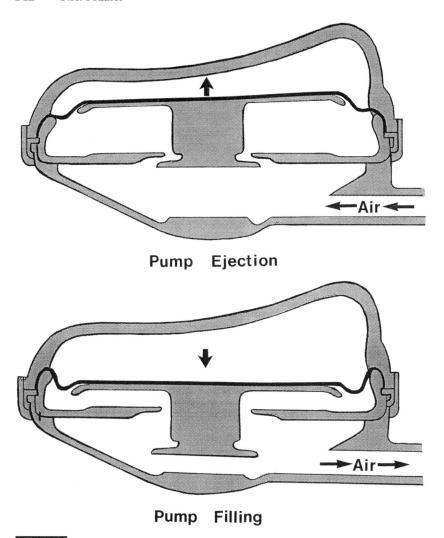

Pump   Ejection

Pump   Filling

FIGURE 4.

As air enters the air chamber of the Implantable Pneumatic left ventricular assist system (IP-LVAS), the diaphragm is forced upward, causing pressurization of the blood chamber. At the completion of pump ejection, the air pressure is released and the pump fills passively. (Courtesy of Myers TJ, Macris MP: Clinical experience with the HeartMate left ventricular assist device. *Heart Failure* 10:247–258, 1994. By permission of *Heart Failure*.)

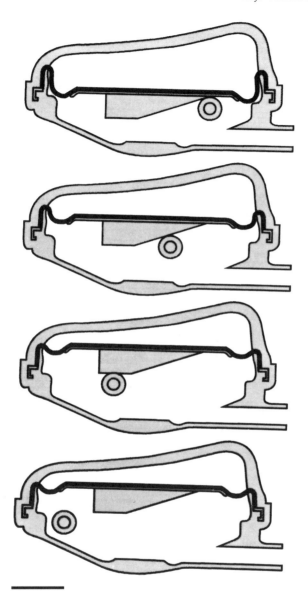

FIGURE 5.

The Vented Electric left ventricular assist system. As the rotor spins, a pair of ball bearings push against a pair of helical cams that are attached to the diaphragm, causing the diaphragm to move up. (Courtesy of Myers TJ, Macris MP: Clinical experience with the HeartMate left ventricular assist device. *Heart Failure* 10:247–258, 1994. By permission of *Heart Failure.*)

However, patients are ineligible for support with a long-term device if they have severe right heart failure, a life-threatening illness other than heart disease, irreversible end-organ failure, respiratory insufficiency requiring intubation, unresolved pulmonary emboli, unacceptable psychosocial history, or are older than 70 years.

Irreversible end-organ dysfunction is one of the most difficult of the contraindicating conditions to assess, because in many cases, end-organ failure can be reversed after a period of mechanical circulatory support. Thus it may be appropriate to implant a device earlier in patients who are in danger of irreversible organ failure. In addition, because mechanical circulatory support can often help end-organ recovery, support with an assist device could make such patients better candidates for transplantation.

COMPLICATIONS

Patients implanted with long-term mechanical support devices are susceptible to a number of complications, including right ventricular failure, bleeding, thromboembolic complications, and infections.

Right Ventricular Failure

Right ventricular failure is a common cause of early death after implantation of a mechanical assist device.[23-26] Some patients with this complication may be treated with pulmonary vasodilators.[27] Others, however, may require temporary mechanical support. Patients who require right ventricular support have a lower survival rate than those who require only left ventricular assistance.[28-30] Unfortunately, the probability of right ventricular failure after device implantation cannot usually be predicted.[31]

Bleeding

Bleeding is the most common complication in patients supported with a long-term mechanical assist device.[23-26] The patients who are most likely to have this complication include those with hepatic congestion and failure, prolonged cardiopulmonary bypass times, extensive surgical dissection, multiple cannulation sites, and platelet interaction with the biomaterial surfaces.[32, 33] In many patients with bleeding (22% to 73%), an operation must be performed.[34, 35] To minimize the risk of reoperation, patients must be carefully monitored for signs of bleeding from the moment they reach the ICU.

Thromboembolic Complications

For many years, thromboembolic complications were a major obstacle to the use of ventricular assistance. With such innovations as the textured, blood-contacting surfaces of the HeartMate, however, the risk of thromboembolic complications has decreased significantly in patients supported with mechanical assist devices.

Infection

Infections are another major complication occurring in patients receiving long-term mechanical circulatory support. Because the current long-term devices all have at least one percutaneous drive line, patients are susceptible to infections at the transcutaneous exit sites.[36] In the HeartMate, the risk of infection is somewhat reduced by the tissue that encapsulates the pump, but the development of completely implantable devices may be the only means of reducing the rate of infection in such patients.

RESULTS

All three devices have been used extensively during the past decade, and all three have had good results. In one multicenter study of the Thoratec, 64% of patients implanted with the Thoratec lived to transplantation. Of the patients who underwent transplantation, 83% survived long term,[17] a rate close to the 82.5% of patients surviving transplantation without circulatory support.[37]

Sixty percent of patients supported with the Novacor LVAS have undergone successful transplantation. Of these patients, 82% were long-term survivors.[22] Again, these percentages are comparable to those of patients receiving transplantation without having been supported by a mechanical assist device.

Between 1986 and 1995, the HeartMate IP-LVAS was implanted in 422 patients around the world.[38] In the FDA trial, 71% of the patients supported with a HeartMate underwent transplantation; however, only 36% of the control patients underwent transplantation. Of these trial patients, 60% of those supported with the HeartMate survived to 60 days, whereas only 30% of the control patients survived to 60 days.[39]

CONCLUSION

What does the future of cardiac assistance have in store for us? Almost certainly, assist devices will become even more prominent fixtures of cardiac treatment. Experimental axial flow pumps such as the Jarvik-2000 will be used routinely in the treatment of patients with chronic heart failure. Long-term pulsatile pumps will be used widely as alternatives to heart transplantation. Finally, pulsatile pumps may be used as bridges to recovery: after a patient's heart has recovered sufficiently, the device will be removed and the patient treated medically. The promise of this technology warrants further testing of these ideas.

REFERENCES

1. Dixon JF, Farris CD, Kimble Jett G: ABIOMED BVS 5000 assist device, in Quaal SJ (ed): *Cardiac Mechanical Assistance Beyond Balloon Pumping.* St Louis, Mosby, 1993, pp 129–143.
2. Shook BJ: The ABIOMED BVS 5000 biventricular support system: System description and clinical summary. *Cardiac Surg: State Art Rev* 7:309–316, 1993.
3. Jett GK: ABIOMED BVS 5000: Experience and potential advantages. *Ann Thorac Surg* 61:301–304, 1996.
4. Guyton RA, Schonberger JP, Everts PA, et al: Postcardiotomy shock: Clinical evaluation of the BVS 5000 biventricular support system. *Ann Thorac Surg* 56:346–356, 1993.
5. Dixon CM, Magovern GJ: Evaluation of the Biopump for long-term cardiac support without heparinization. *J Extracorporeal Technology* 14:331–336, 1982.
6. Joyce LD, Toninato C, Hansen JB: Centrifugal ventricular assist devices, in Quaal SJ (ed): *Cardiac Mechanical Assistance Beyond Balloon Pumping.* St Louis, Mosby, 1993, pp 55–66.
7. Frazier OH: New technologies in the treatment of severe cardiac failure: The Texas Heart Institute experience. *Ann Thorac Surg* 59:S31–S38, 1995.
8. Noon GP: Bio-Medicus ventricular assistance (editorial). *Ann Thorac Surg* 52:180–181, 1991.
9. Killen DA, Piehler JM, Borkon AM, et al: Bio-Medicus ventricular assist device for salvage of cardiac surgical patients. *Ann Thorac Surg* 52:230–235, 1991.
10. Golding LA, Stewart RW, Sinkewich M, et al: Nonpulsatile ventricular assist bridging to transplantation. *ASAIO Trans* 34:476–479, 1988.
11. Golding LA: The development and clinical use of centrifugal blood pumps, in Lewis T, Graham TR (eds): *Mechanical Circulatory Support.* London, Edward Arnold, 1995, pp 153–158.
12. Wampler RK, Moise JC, Frazier OH, et al: In vivo evaluation of a peripheral vascular access axial flow blood pump. *ASAIO Trans* 34:450–454, 1988.
13. Wampler RK: The development and future of the Hemopump, in Lewis T, Graham TR (eds): *Mechanical Circulatory Support.* London, Edward Arnold, 1995, pp 136–145.
14. Frazier OH, Wampler RK, Duncan JM, et al: First human use of the Hemopump, a catheter-mounted ventricular assist device. *Ann Thorac Surg* 49:299–304, 1990.
15. Merhige ME, Smalling RW, Cassidy D, et al: Effect of the Hemopump left ventricular assist device on regional myocardial perfusion and function. Reduction of ischemia during coronary occlusion. *Circulation* 80:158S–166S, 1989.

16. Wampler RK, Frazier OH, Lansing AM, et al: Treatment of cardiogenic shock with the Hemopump left ventricular assist device. *Ann Thorac Surg* 52:506–513, 1991.

17. Hill JD, Farrar DJ: The Thoratec VAD System: Patient selection and clinical results in bridging to transplantation, in Lewis T, Graham TR (eds): *Mechanical Circulatory Support.* London, Edward Arnold, 1995, pp 169–175.

18. Frazier OH: Long-term mechanical circulatory support, in Edmunds LH Jr (ed): *Cardiac Surgery in the Adult.* New York, McGraw-Hill, (in press.)

19. Farrar DJ, Hill JD, Gray LA Jr, et al: Heterotopic prosthetic ventricles as a bridge to cardiac transplantation. A multicenter study in 29 patients. *N Engl J Med* 318:333–340, 1988.

20. Frazier OH, Short HD, Wampler RK, et al: Mechanical circulatory support in the transplant population, in Frazier OH (ed): *Support and Replacement of the Failing Heart.* Philadelphia, Lippincott-Raven, 1996, pp 147–167.

21. Burnett CM, Duncan JM, Frazier OH, et al: Improved multiorgan function after prolonged univentricular support. *Ann Thorac Surg* 55:65–71, 1993.

22. Pennington DG, Portner PM, Swartz MT: Clinical experience with the Novacor left ventricular assist system, in Lewis T, Graham TR (eds): *Mechanical Circulatory Support.* London, Edward Arnold, 1995, pp 225–228.

23. Shinn JA: Novacor left ventricular assist system. *AACN Clinical Issues in Critical Care Nursing* 2:575–586, 1991.

24. Korfer R, El-Banayosy A, Posival H, et al: Mechanical circulatory support: The Bad Oeynhausen experience. *Ann Thorac Surg* 59:S56–S62, 1995.

25. Frazier OH, Rose EA, McCarthy P, et al: Improved mortality and rehabilitation of transplant candidates treated with a long-term implantable left ventricular assist system. *Ann Surg* 222:327–336, 1995.

26. Mehta SM, Aufiero TX, Pae WE Jr, et al: Combined registry for the clinical use of mechanical ventricular assist pumps and the total artificial heart in conjunction with heart transplantation: Sixth official report—1994. *J Heart Lung Transplant* 14:585–593, 1995.

27. D'Ambra MN, LaRaia PJ, Philbin DM, et al: Prostaglandin E_1. A new therapy for refractory right heart failure and pulmonary hypertension after mitral valve replacement. *J Thorac Cardiovasc Surg* 89:567–572, 1985.

28. Farrar DJ, Hill JD: Univentricular and biventricular Thoratec VAD support as a bridge to transplantation. *Ann Thorac Surg* 55:276–282, 1993.

29. Portner PM, Oyer PE, Pennington DG, et al: Implantable electrical left ventricular assist system: Bridge to transplantation and the future. *Ann Thorac Surg* 47:142–150, 1989.

30. Frazier OH, Rose EA, Macmanus Q, et al: Multicenter clinical evaluation of the HeartMate 1000 IP left ventricular assist device. *Ann Thorac Surg* 53:1080–1090, 1992.

31. Kormos RL, Borovetz HS, Gasior T, et al: Experience with univentricular support in mortally ill cardiac transplant candidates. *Ann Thorac Surg* 49:261–271, 1990.
32. Shinn JA, Oyer PE: Novacor ventricular assist system, in Quaal SJ (ed): *Cardiac Mechanical Assistance Beyond Balloon Pumping.* St Louis, Mosby, 1993, pp 99–115.
33. Farrar DJ, Lawson JH, Litwak P, et al: Thoratec VAD system as a bridge to heart transplantation. *J Heart Lung Transplant* 9:415–422, 1990.
34. Pennington DG, Kanter KR, McBride LR, et al: Seven years' experience with the Pierce-Donachy ventricular assist device. *J Thorac Cardiovasc Surg* 96:901–911, 1988.
35. Reedy JE, Ruzevich SA, Noedel NR, et al: Nursing care of the ambulatory patient with a mechanical assist device. *J Heart Lung Transplant* 9:97–105, 1990.
36. Pennington DG, Swartz MT: Infectious complications associated with ventricular assist device support, in Lewis T, Graham TR (eds): *Mechanical Circulatory Support.* London, Edward Arnold, 1995, pp 322–326.
37. Pifarre R, Sullivan H, Montoya A, et al: Comparison of results after heart transplantation: Mechanically supported versus nonsupported patients. *J Heart Lung Transplant* 11:235–239, 1992.
38. Myers TJ, Dasse KA, Macris MP, et al: Use of a left ventricular assist device in an outpatient setting. *ASAIO J* 40:M471–M475, 1994.
39. Frazier OH, Rose EA, McCarthy P, et al: Improved mortality and rehabilitation of transplant candidates treated with a long-term implantable left ventricular assist system. *Ann Surg* 222:327–336, 1995.

CHAPTER 9

Pediatric Cardiac Transplantation

David C. McGiffin, M.D.
Associate Professor, Department of Surgery, Division of Cardiothoracic
Surgery, University of Alabama, Birmingham, Alabama

James K. Kirklin, M.D.
Professor, Department of Surgery, Division of Cardiothoracic Surgery,
University of Alabama, Birmingham, Alabama

F. Bennett Pearce, M.D.
Assistant Professor, Department of Pediatrics, Division of Pediatric
Cardiology, University of Alabama, Birmingham, Alabama

C ardiac transplantation for infants and children is now established therapy, but the road traveled to reach this position has
been paved with many disappointments. Fortunately, the advances
made in adult cardiac transplantation have directly impacted on
cardiac transplantation in children. Because of this, together with
progress in the aspects peculiar to pediatric transplantation such
as the surgical details in patients with complex congenital heart
disease, the diagnosis of acute cardiac rejection in infants, and protocols for maintaining neonates before transplantation, the results
have steadily improved. One of the important challenges in pediatric cardiac transplantation is to define its role in the overall management of a variety of unfavorable congenital and acquired heart
diseases in infants and children, with the purpose of developing a
patient-specific therapeutic strategy to provide a child with the best
possible duration and quality of life. Of course, cardiac transplantation should be considered as a course of therapy because the truly
long-term results of cardiac transplantation in children are unknown, and it is likely that more than one transplant will be required because of the subsequent appearance of coronary allograft
vasculopathy.

This chapter reviews the history of pediatric cardiac transplantation, recipient selection, donor selection, surgical details,

Advances in Cardiac Surgery®, vol. 9
© 1997, Mosby–Year Book, Inc.

immunosuppression, and results of cardiac transplantation in children.

HISTORY

The first report of a cardiac transplant in a child was by Kantrowitz et al., who performed an orthotopic cardiac transplant procedure on an infant aged 18 days with Ebstein's malformation, refractory congestive heart failure, and a previous aortopulmonary shunt.[1] This procedure occurred 3 days after the first human-to-human heart transplant in 1967. The patient received a heart from an anencephalic infant and died 5 hours after the procedure. Cooley et al. performed the first cardiopulmonary transplant in 1968[2] in an infant 2 months of age with an atrioventricular septal defect, but the infant died 14 hours after the procedure. Subsequent attempts at cardiac transplantation in infants and children during the next 20 years were sporadic with poor results. With the progressive improvement in the results of cardiac transplantation in adults, there was renewed interest in transplantation in children. In 1985, Yacoub and Radley-Smith opened the way for transplantation in neonates by performing a transplant in a patient with hypoplastic left heart syndrome[3]: the baby died 23 days after the procedure of necrotizing enterocolitis. However, it was the seminal work of Bailey and colleagues[4] at Loma Linda that established cardiac transplantation as a viable option for hypoplastic left heart syndrome. Bailey and colleagues were also responsible for a much publicized foray into xenotransplantation[5]—the "Baby Fae" experiment in which a baboon heart was transplanted into a newborn infant with hypoplastic left heart syndrome in 1984, with the baby surviving 20 days. This, not surprisingly, resulted in vigorous public debate regarding the issue of primate donors for human transplantation.

RECIPIENT SELECTION

There are four general categories of disease processes in which cardiac transplantation can be considered as a therapeutic option. Obviously, the indications for cardiac transplantation in children are still in evolution, and the place of transplantation, particularly for children with congenital heart disease, should be considered in the context of progress in the correction of complex congenital heart disease. In these children the concept of a "therapeutic strategy" that involves cardiac transplantation should be considered, which may incorporate one or more palliative procedures followed by cardiac transplantation (during a lifetime may involve more than one transplant). These four general categories include (1) cardiomyopathic processes, (2) anatomically uncorrectable congenital heart disease, (3) refractory heart failure after previous surgery for congenital heart disease, and (4) rare indications such as cardiac tumors.

CARDIOMYOPATHY IN CHILDHOOD

Cardiomyopathy refers to a group of disorders defined by the World Health Organization/International Society and Federation of Cardiologists as a disease of heart muscle that is not secondary to an acquired or congenital heart disease.[6] There are three patterns that are usually described. *Dilated cardiomyopathy* is characterized by left or biventricular systolic dysfunction and dilatation. The clinical syndrome is usually congestive heart failure that may include important atrial and ventricular arrhythmias. *Hypertrophic cardiomyopathy* is characterized by inappropriate left ventricular hypertrophy with preserved ventricular systolic function and often a left ventricular outflow tract gradient. The presentation and course are usually characterized by dyspnea, chest pain, and arrhythmias, and it is an important cause of sudden death in young adults and athletes. This condition is not usually seen with symptoms of congestive heart failure. *Restrictive cardiomyopathy* is rare in children and is characterized by biventricular diastolic dysfunction with marked atrial enlargement. Symptoms result from systemic and pulmonary venous congestion.

In a study by Chen and colleagues, the 1- and 5-year mortality rates for children with dilated cardiomyopathy were 30% and 44%, respectively, but are highly dependent on the type and severity of the pathologic process.[7] A study of 24 patients younger than 2 years who were seen at the Boston Children's Hospital between 1982 and 1990 demonstrated a mortality of 30%, with all deaths except one occurring within 2 months of presentation.[8] Similarly, a study from the Mayo Clinic demonstrated a 1-year mortality rate of 37% and a 5-year mortality rate of 66%.[9] A number of factors have been identified that are generally associated with poor survival, including older age at presentation[10] (5–15 years vs. younger than 2 years of age at presentation), persistent congestive heart failure,[11] echocardiographic pattern of low shortening fraction,[7] and the presence of endocardial fibroelastosis.[7] The development of complex atrial and ventricular arrhythmias as a risk factor for death remains controversial.[10, 11]

Three special cardiomyopathic processes for which cardiac transplantation may be considered include myocarditis, disorders of metabolism, and adriamycin toxicity. However, evidence exists that the natural history of acute dilated cardiomyopathy associated with myocarditis may be favorably affected by the administration of IV γ-globulin,[12] and hence transplantation may either be delayed or not required.

The clinical course of hypertrophic cardiomyopathy is variable and unpredictable. The natural history of this process may be favorably influenced by medical therapy, implantation of a permanent pacing system, or relief of left ventricular outflow tract obstruction. The annual mortality rate for children with hypertrophic cardiomyopathy appears to be 4% to 6%.[13]

The clinical course of restrictive cardiomyopathy in children is not well documented, but the natural history of the disease appears poor. A study by Lewis indicates that the probability of surviving 4 years after the diagnosis of restrictive cardiomyopathy is 29%.[14]

Despite these survival and risk factor data, it should be noted that rigorous natural history studies and risk factor analyses are largely unavailable for childhood cardiomyopathies. Therefore, the precise indications for cardiac transplantation have not yet been clearly determined.

ANATOMICALLY UNCORRECTABLE CONGENITAL HEART DISEASE

There are a number of congenital cardiac defects, particularly those characterized by severe underdevelopment of one ventricle, for which a two-ventricular repair is not possible. For these patients, a pathway leading to the Fontan procedure is the only surgical option currently available. Hypoplastic left heart syndrome, the condition for which the largest proportion of infants undergo transplantation in the first year of life,[4] may be treated by a series of palliative procedures (Norwood operation) leading to a modified Fontan procedure, but the results vary considerably. A few institutions have obtained good short- and intermediate-term survival, but for most institutions, short-term and midterm mortality is high. A number of other institutions have adopted cardiac transplantation as the treatment of choice, but because of the shortage of donor hearts and the progressive improvement of the results of the Norwood procedure, there is currently no clear survival advantage of one therapy over another. A number of other forms of anatomically uncorrectable congenital heart disease that can be considered for cardiac transplantation include pulmonary atresia with intact ventricular septum with marked coronary sinusoids, interrupted aortic arch with severe left ventricular outflow tract obstruction, complete atrioventricular septal defects with severe right or left ventricular dominance, and complex single ventricle with asplenia. For patients with these conditions for whom the traditional approach has been the Fontan operation but who may have risk factors associated with a poor result after the Fontan procedure (moderately small pulmonary arteries, atrioventricular valve insufficiency or impaired systemic ventricular function), cardiac transplantation may be the procedure of choice.

HEART FAILURE AFTER PREVIOUS SURGERY FOR CONGENITAL HEART DISEASE

After surgery for complex congenital heart disease, a number of patients may subsequently have indications for cardiac transplantation develop. The two most common indications are failure of the Fontan procedure (as evidenced by recurrent ascites, generalized fluid retention, and low systemic cardiac output) and refractory systemic ventricular failure after two ventricle repairs. For this latter group of patients, the same medical therapy and decision making regarding timing of cardiac transplantation apply as for adult patients.

RARE INDICATIONS

Although rare, there are infants and children who may require cardiac transplantation for unresectable cardiac tumors and other diseases such as Kawasaki's disease.

In the series of infants undergoing cardiac transplantation in the first year of life from Loma Linda,[4] the great majority of procedures were for hypoplastic left heart syndrome, although a number of patients had complex lesions such as unbalanced atrioventricular septal defect, pulmonary atresia with intact ventricular septum with right ventricular dependent coronary circulation, right or left atrial isomerism, and complex lesions associated with left ventricular outflow tract obstruction. Included in this study were also patients with dilated cardiomyopathy, and of particular interest, two patients undergoing transplantation for cardiac tumors. In a series of patients undergoing cardiac transplantation who were older than 1 year (obtained from the multicenter Pediatric Heart Transplant Study),[15] 39% underwent transplantation for idiopathic dilated cardiomyopathy, 38% for complex congenital heart disease, 7% for myocarditis, 5% for hypertrophic cardiomyopathy, 5% for restrictive cardiomyopathy, 3% for adriamycin cardiomyopathy, and a small percentage of patients for other conditions such as ischemic cardiomyopathy, acquired valvular heart disease, and cardiac tumors.

The selection of infants and children for cardiac transplantation requires consideration of many of the same factors involved in the selection of adults for cardiac transplantation, with the exception that in infants and children with complex uncorrectable heart disease (and patients with correctable heart disease who are at an increased operative risk), the likelihood of success with conventional corrective procedures must be part of the decision-making process. For children with cardiomyopathic processes whose symptoms may not be marked, the timing of cardiac transplantation must take into account the natural history of the disease.

The contraindications to cardiac transplantation that are peculiar to pediatric patients are largely anatomical ones; they principally relate to abnormalities of the pulmonary arteries, which include small pulmonary arteries (the lower limit of pulmonary artery size that would preclude transplantation is unknown), and abnormalities of peripheral pulmonary arborization to a degree that would predict a right ventricular systolic pressure exceeding approximately 50–55 mm Hg at the conclusion of the transplant procedure. Abnormalities of pulmonary venous return in which a connection between pulmonary veins and the left atrium cannot be made would also preclude cardiac transplantation. Elevation of pulmonary vascular resistance poses the same concerns in pediatric patients as in adult patients, although in infants the use of strategies such as nitric oxide inhalation therapy[16] may ameliorate the progression of pulmonary vascular disease in neonates at risk from this process who are awaiting cardiac transplantation.

OUTCOME AFTER LISTING FOR CARDIAC TRANSPLANTATION

The decision regarding the appropriateness of cardiac transplantation for a patient is made either formally or informally by comparing the survival after cardiac transplantation with either the natural history of the disease process (e.g., dilated cardiomyopathy) or the survival after conventional surgery in the case of complex congenital heart disease. Because a potential source of mortality occurs between the time of listing and the performance of cardiac transplantation, any analysis of survival after cardiac transplantation needs to include the waiting time before transplant.

By studying outcomes of patients after listing for pediatric cardiac transplantation, important information regarding the appropriateness of listing of patients with certain cardiac diseases, as well as the availability and allocation of donor organs, can be gained. However, it is important that the appropriate statistical tools are applied to the analysis of outcomes after listing for cardiac transplantation. The traditional method of analyzing time-related events such as outcomes after listing for transplantation is the Kaplan-Meier estimate,[17] which was originally devised to portray a single time-related event. Analysis of outcome after listing for pediatric cardiac transplantation is complicated by the multiple outcomes that are possible after listing: (1) removal from the list because of change in clinical condition (improving or worsening), (2) death while waiting for transplantation, (3) transplantation, and (4) continuing to wait for transplantation. Consequently, because of the censoring process in the situation of multiple competing events, a Kaplan-Meier method may produce an inaccurate estimate of the proportion of patients actually experiencing an event after listing.

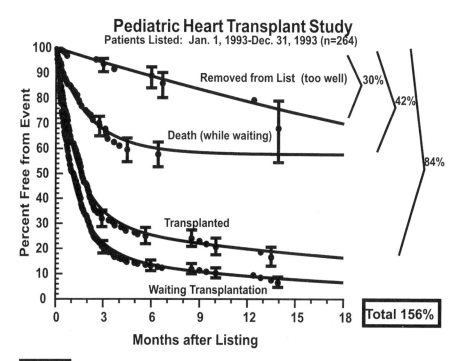

FIGURE 1.

Parametric estimate *(solid lines)* and Kaplan-Meier depiction *(dots)* of the freedom from removal from the list (too well), death while waiting, transplantation, and waiting for transplantation with the 70% confidence limits *(vertical bars).* Because of the censoring process, the sum of the probabilities of each event is greater than 100%. (Courtesy of McGiffin DC, Naftel DC, Kirklin JK, et al: Predicting outcome following listing for cardiac transplantation in children: Comparison of Kaplan-Meier and parametric competing risk analysis. *J Heart Lung Transplant,* in press.)

McGiffin and colleagues[18] studied the outcome of 264 patients after listing for pediatric cardiac transplantation. The Kaplan-Meier depiction of each possible outcome is depicted in Figure 1. Note that the sum of the possible outcomes in the Kaplan-Meier analysis at any point in time exceeds 1.0. Therefore, the Kaplan-Meier method answers the question, "What is the probability of a particular event provided there is no opportunity for any other event to occur?". However, the question that is of most interest is, "What is the probability of actually experiencing one of these events?".

The answer to this question is provided by the competing outcomes method and simultaneously solves for all possible outcomes. Figure 2 depicts the actual proportion of patients experiencing any of the possible outcomes after listing. At any point in time from listing, the sum of the proportions of patients actually

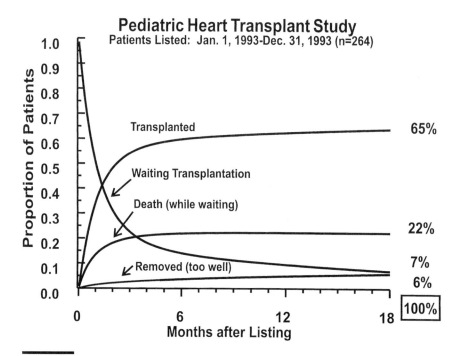

FIGURE 2.

Parametric estimates of proportion of patients *actually* transplanted, dying while waiting, removed from the list (too well), and waiting for transplantation. Using the competing outcomes method, the sum of the probabilities of each event is 100%. (Courtesy of McGiffin DC, Naftel DC, Kirklin JK, et al: Predicting outcome following listing for cardiac transplantation in children: Comparison of Kaplan-Meier and parametric competing risk analysis. *J Heart Lung Transplant,* in press.)

experiencing each outcome is 100%. The incorporation of patient-specific predictions in the competing outcomes analysis can also provide further insights. The risk factors associated with each of the possible outcomes after listing (by multivariable analyses) are shown in Table 1. It is interesting to examine the probability of each of the possible outcomes for two patients with different risk factor profiles. The probability of each of the outcome events for patient 1 (United Network of Organ Sharing [UNOS] status 1, 1 month of age, receiving mechanical ventilation, blood group A, negative cytomegalovirus [CMV] serologic testing) is depicted in Figure 3. The fate of this patient was determined relatively rapidly after listing. In contrast, the probability of each of the outcome events in a patient with a risk factor profile of patient 2 (UNOS status 2, 10 years of age, blood group O, positive CMV serologic testing) is extremely different in that the process of "assortment" into the various possible outcomes is occurring at a far slower rate than that of patient 1 (Fig 4). This type of analysis is important because the Kaplan-Meier estimate can be misunderstood and could, for example, suggest (see Fig 1) that an important number of patients are being in-

TABLE 1.
Risk Factors for Outcomes

Longer Time to Transplantation		Death While Waiting		Remove From List (Too Well)	
Infants	**Children**	**Infants**	**Children**	**Infants**	**Children**
HLHS					
	Status 2	Inotropic support	Status 1	None Identified	
Smaller size	Blood type O	Smaller size	Ventilator		
Blood type O	Positive CMV	Blood type O			
Non-HLHS					
Younger age					

Abbreviations: HLHS, hypoplastic left heart syndrome; *CMV*, cytomegalovirus.
(Courtesy of McGiffin DC, Naftel DC, Kirklin JK, et al: Predicting outcome following listing for cardiac transplantation in children: Comparison of Kaplan-Meier and parametric competing risk analysis. *J Heart Lung Transplant*, in press.)

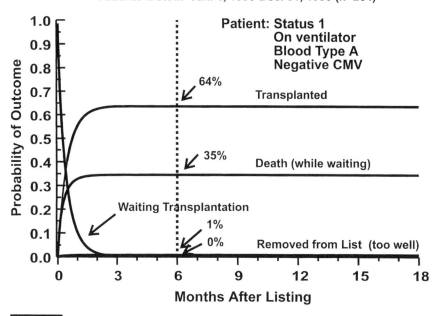

Pediatric Heart Transplant Study
Patients Listed: Jan. 1, 1993-Dec. 31, 1993 (n=264)

FIGURE 3.

Predicted parametric estimates in the competing risk domain of each of the possible outcomes after listing for a patient with the characteristics of patient 1. (Courtesy of McGiffin DC, Naftel DC, Kirklin JK, et al: Predicting outcome following listing for cardiac transplantation in children: Comparison of Kaplan-Meier and parametric competing risk analysis. *J Heart Lung Transplant,* in press.)

appropriately listed for transplantation when they have the potential for improvement, but the competing risk analysis (see Fig 2) indicates that this is not the case. The incorporation of patient-specific predictions in the competing outcomes analysis can be used in a practical sense to optimize the time of individual patient listing for transplantation.

DONOR SELECTION

The diagnosis of brain death in infants and children has been controversial, and for that reason the original criteria established for determining brain death in adults were not extended to children younger than 5 years,[19] resulting from concerns[20] about the accuracy of the diagnosis of brain death. For example, the brains of newborns tend to be less vulnerable to asphyxial injury than the brains

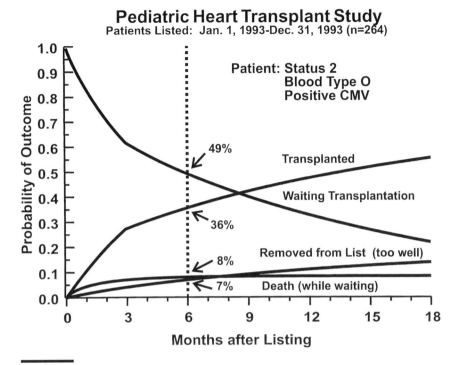

Pediatric Heart Transplant Study
Patients Listed: Jan. 1, 1993-Dec. 31, 1993 (n=264)

Patient: Status 2
Blood Type O
Positive CMV

49%

Transplanted

Waiting Transplantation

36%

Removed from List (too well)

8%

7%   Death (while waiting)

Months after Listing

FIGURE 4.

Predicted parametric estimates in the competing risk domain of each of the possible outcomes after listing for a patient with the characteristics of patient 2. (Courtesy of McGiffin DC, Naftel DC, Kirklin JK, et al: Predicting outcome following listing for cardiac transplantation in children: Comparison of Kaplan-Meier and parametric competing risk analysis. *J Heart Lung Transplant,* in press.)

of older infants and children, phenobarbital is often used in the treatment of seizures associated with perinatal asphyxia, neurologic developmental abnormalities may complicate the diagnosis of brain death, and hypotension may significantly decrease cerebral blood flow in preterm and term infants. Despite these concerns, the diagnosis of brain death in preterm and term infants can usually be made clinically, and current guidelines include a period of observation because of these confounding factors.[20]

The causes of brain death in infant donors[4] often differ from those in children and adults and include birth asphyxia, sudden infant death syndrome, metabolic causes, intracanial hemorrhage, infection, and child abuse, whereas the causes of brain death in children[21] include predominantly trauma (penetrating and nonpenetrating) and rarer events such as intracranial hemorrhage and smoke inhalation.

The general contraindications to infant heart donation are (1) complex cardiac malformation, (2) overwhelming untreated sepsis, (3) suspected hepatitis or retrovirus infection, and (4) marked reduction in myocardial contractility after appropriate volume loading and inotropic support (with a fractional shortening of less than 25% and/or major wall motion abnormalities).[4] The issue of the dysfunctional neonatal donor heart is important because donor myocardial dysfunction may be reversible. A study by Boucek et al. found that neonatal donor hearts with decreased left ventricular function (left ventricular shortening fraction of 0.15–0.28 and/or segmental wall motion abnormalities) can function normally in the recipient.[22] No difference in early mortality was observed in the group of patients receiving a dysfunctional donor heart vs. those receiving a normally functioning heart. Infant donor hearts from patients who have undergone extended CPR (up to 2 hours) have also been successfully used for transplantation by the Loma Linda group[23] provided the shortening fraction by echocardiography was at least 0.14 and inotropic support did not exceed 20 μ/kg per minute of dopamine and/or dobutamine or 0.2 μg/kg per minute of epinephrine. These donor hearts were procured from 18 hours to 4 days after CPR. It is interesting that in this group of patients, the hemodynamics within the first week after transplantation were normal, and there was no mortality in the recipients receiving these hearts. It seems reasonable then to extend donor criteria so that donor hearts that would have been traditionally regarded as very marginal for transplantation can be used.

Donor-recipient size matching is important, yet incomplete information is available about the limits of mismatching in infants and children. Based on a study by Fullerton et al.,[24] it would appear that a disparate donor-recipient weight mismatch ratio (approximately 0.5–3.0) can be tolerated without increasing perioperative mortality. Unfortunately, others have not had the same experience, and Tamisier and colleagues[25] have, on the basis of their experience, cautioned against accepting a donor-recipient weight ratio of less than one.

A variety of preservation solutions have been used for infant cardiac transplantation, but available experimental evidence suggests better preservation with University of Wisconsin solution compared with extracellular cardioplegic solutions. The neonatal myocardium may possibly be less vulnerable to ischemic and hypoxemic injury than adult myocardium, and successful infant cardiac transplantation has been reported with ischemic times up to 10 hours with a variety of preservation solutions. Kawauchi and colleagues from Loma Linda found no relationship between the duration of ischemic time (maximum, 8 hours 2 minutes) and the probability of primary graft failure,[26] although there was evidence of diastolic dysfunction (disappeared in the second postoperative week) with longer ischemic times. The method of preservation was Roe's solution, an acalcemic solution with a high concentration of glucose.

SURGICAL TECHNIQUES

Cardiac transplantation in infants and children is frequently associated with greater surgical complexity than that in adults because of associated congenital heart disease. Congenital malformations that require technical modifications include hypoplastic left heart syndrome, single atrium, anomalies of systemic or pulmonary venous return, transposition or malposition of the great vessels, pre-

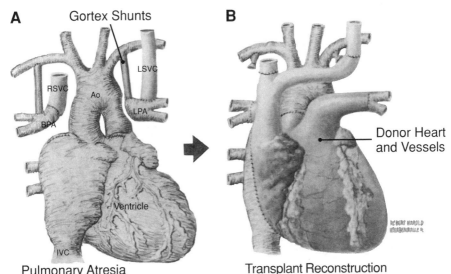

A, Gortex Shunts — LSVC, RSVC, Ao, LPA, RPA, Ventricle, IVC

Pulmonary Atresia
Bilateral Systemic-Pulmonary Shunts
Bilateral Cavopulmonary Shunts

B, Donor Heart and Vessels

Transplant Reconstruction

FIGURE 5.
A, Pathologic anatomy of recipient subjected to multiple palliative interventions that ended in cavopulmonary shunts and destroyed central pulmonary arteries. **B,** final appearance of heart transplant in the same patient. *Abbreviations: Ao,* aorta, *IVC,* inferior vena cava; *LPA,* left pulmonary artery; *LSVC,* left superior vena cava; *LPA,* left pulmonary artery; *RSVC,* right superior vena cava; *RPA,* right pulmonary artery. (Courtesy of Bailey LL: Heart transplantation techniques in complex congenital heart disease. *J Heart Lung Transplant* 12:168S–175S, 1993.)

vious atrial septation operation, situs inversus, cavopulmonary shunts, aortopulmonary shunts, and absent or deficient central pulmonary arteries.

Technical variations may be required for donor cardiectomy because of recipient congenital heart anomalies. For example, where the heart is to be transplanted for hypoplastic left heart syndrome, the donor heart must be excised together with the entire aortic arch and upper descending thoracic aorta after division of the inominate, left carotid, and left subclavian arteries. Other technical variations include procurement of the left and right pulmonary arteries where pulmonary artery reconstruction in the recipient is required (Figs 5 and 6).[27]

For recipients without complicating congenital cardiac anomalies, the standard technique of Lower and Shumway is used.

Implantation of the donor heart in patients with hypoplastic left heart syndrome is based on the original technique described by Bailey et al.[28] The procedure is performed using cardiopulmonary bypass with double or single venous cannulation, profound hypothermia to 20° C, and circulatory arrest either for the entire implant procedure or limited to reconstruction of the aortic arch

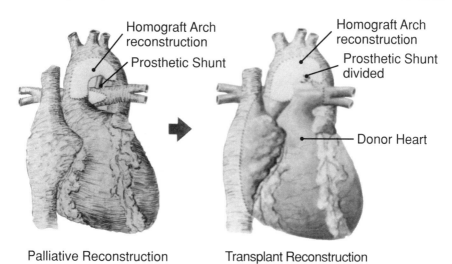

Homograft Arch reconstruction

Prosthetic Shunt

Homograft Arch reconstruction

Prosthetic Shunt divided

Donor Heart

Palliative Reconstruction   Transplant Reconstruction

FIGURE 6.

Completed but failed stage I Norwood reconstruction before and after secondary heart transplantation. Note reconstruction of central pulmonary arteries by en bloc donor pulmonary artery. (Courtesy of Bailey LL: Heart transplantation techniques in complex congenital heart disease. *J Heart Lung Transplant* 12:168S–175S, 1993.)

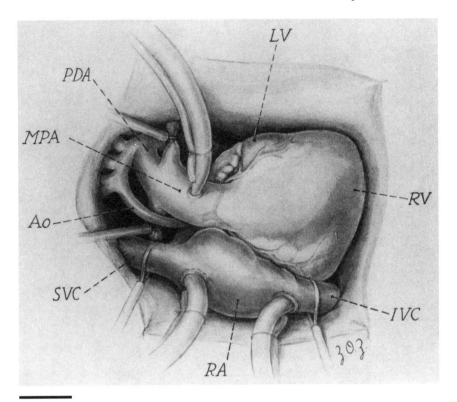

FIGURE 7.
Cannulation for orthotopic cardiac transplantation in an infant with hypoplastic left heart syndrome (type I). Arterial perfusion is via an 8F catheter in the main pulmonary artery *(MPA)*. Note snares around right and left pulmonary arteries to prevent flow to the lungs. Venous return is with bicaval cannulation, 12F cannula in the superior vena cava *(SVC)* and 16F cannula in the inferior vena cava *(IVC)*. Abbreviations: *Ao,* aorta; *LV,* left ventricle; *PDA,* patent ductus arteriosus; *RA,* right atrium; *RV,* right ventricle. (Courtesy of Backer CL, Idriss FS, Zales VR, et al: Cardiac transplantation for hypoplastic left heart syndrome: A modified technique, *Ann Thorac Surg* 50:894–898, 1990. Reprinted with permission from the Society of Thoracic Surgeons.)

(Figs 7 and 8).[29] The left atrial anastomosis is performed (Fig 9)[29] followed by reconstruction of the aortic arch (Figs 10 and 11),[29] after which the right atrial and pulmonary artery anastomoses are constricted (Fig 12).[29]

IMMUNOSUPPRESSION

If cardiac transplantation is performed within the first few days or weeks of postnatal life, the probability of acute cardiac rejection

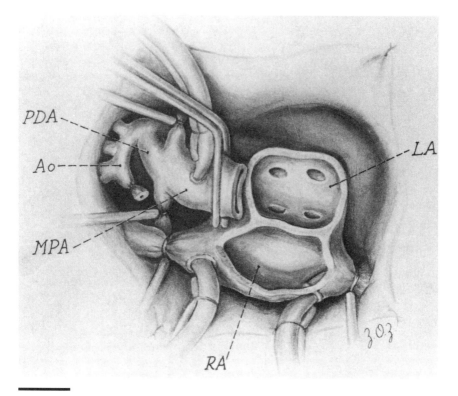

FIGURE 8.

The heart has been excised after placement of a cross-clamp on the main pulmonary artery *(MPA)* and ligation and division of the tiny ascending aorta *(Ao)*. Excision of the donor heart is performed with extracorporeal circulation continuing. *Abbreviations: LA,* left atrium; *PDA,* patent ductus arteriosus; *RA,* right atrium. (Courtesy of Backer CL, Idriss FS, Zales VR, et al: Cardiac transplantation for hypoplastic left heart syndrome: A modified technique, *Ann Thorac Surg* 50:894–898, 1990. Reprinted with permission from the Society of Thoracic Surgeons.)

may be less than in older infants despite relatively low doses of immunosuppressive agents ("window of opportunity" of neonatal cardiac transplantation).[30] Neonatal hyporesponsiveness has been demonstrated in animals, but amelioration of the immune response in human neonates has not been clearly established.

A number of different immunosuppression protocols are in use, and, to date, any differences in survival cannot be attributed to the variability between protocols. Some transplant centers use induction therapy with either OKT3 or with an antilymphocyte globulin preparation, as well as cyclosporine, azathioprine, and steroids. Maintenance immunosuppression is based on cyclosporine either as double therapy with azathioprine or triple therapy with azathioprine and steroids. The management of cyclosporine therapy differs in infants and children compared with that in adults because of the more rapid hepatic metabolism of the drug, and,

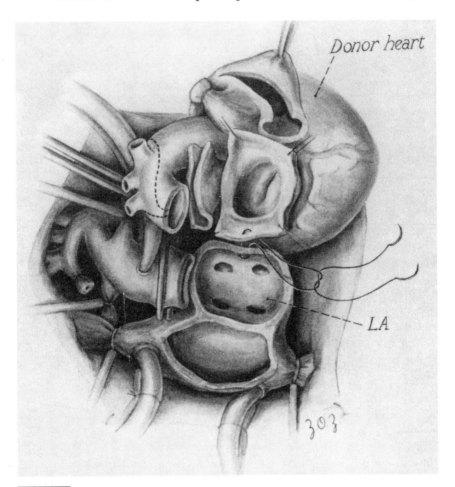

FIGURE 9.
The donor heart is brought into the field, and the left atrial *(LA)* anastomosis is performed while extracorporeal circulation is maintained. The donor arch is tailored as indicated by the *dotted lines.* (Courtesy of Backer CL, Idriss FS, Zales VR, et al: Cardiac transplantation for hypoplastic left heart syndrome: A modified technique, *Ann Thorac Surg* 50:894–898, 1990. Reprinted with permission from the Society of Thoracic Surgeons.)

hence, higher doses given more frequently (three times per day) are required. In some centers, maintenance steroids are not used and steroids are only used for the treatment of acute cardiac rejection.[4] Other centers have made a concerted effort to withdraw steroids after 6–12 months.[31]

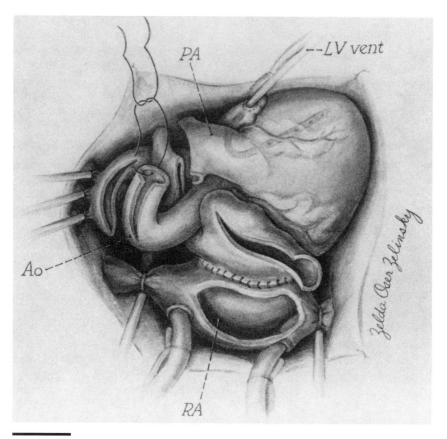

FIGURE 10.

An 8F catheter has been placed in the left ventricle for instillation of cold saline solution. Circulatory arrest is initiated after the head vessels have been controlled by temporary occlusion. The ductus arteriosus is ligated and divided and the main pulmonary artery *(PA)* transected proximal to the bifurcation. The recipient aortic arch is prepared by aortotomy across the transverse arch and coarctation site (distal to the ligated patent ductus arteriosus). *Abbreviations: Ao,* aorta; *LV,* left ventricular; *RA,* right atrium. (Courtesy of Backer CL, Idriss FS, Zales VR, et al: Cardiac transplantation for hypoplastic left heart syndrome: A modified technique, *Ann Thorac Surg* 50:894–898, 1990. Reprinted with permission from the Society of Thoracic Surgeons.)

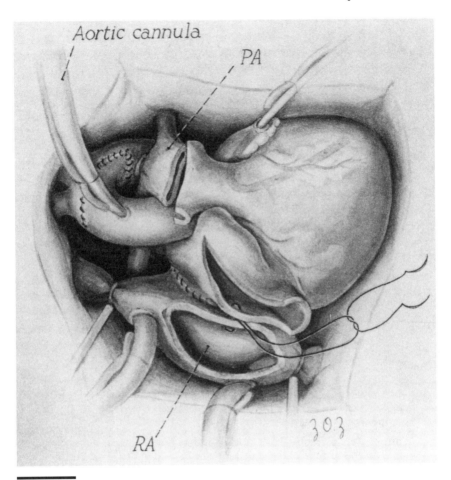

FIGURE 11.

The aortic arch reconstruction is completed, procedures to remove air are performed, and the arch is cannulated (8F), reinstituting cardiopulmonary bypass. The right atrial *(RA)* and the pulmonary artery *(PA)* anastomoses are performed with the heart perfused while the infant is rewarmed. The catheter in the left ventricle is now used as a vent. (Courtesy of Backer CL, Idriss FS, Zales VR, et al: Cardiac transplantation for hypoplastic left heart syndrome: A modified technique, *Ann Thorac Surg* 50:894–898, 1990. Reprinted with permission from the Society of Thoracic Surgeons.)

ACUTE CARDIAC REJECTION

As in adults, the highest incidence of acute cardiac rejection after cardiac transplantation in infants and children is in the first 3–6 postoperative months. The basis for the diagnosis of acute cardiac

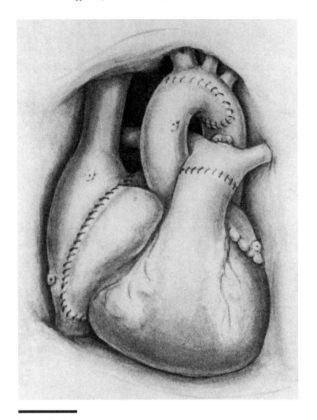

FIGURE 12.

Cardiac transplantation has been completed, and the cannulas have been removed. (Courtesy of Backer CL, Idriss FS, Zales VR, et al: Cardiac transplantation for hypoplastic left heart syndrome: A modified technique, *Ann Thorac Surg* 50:894–898, 1990. Reprinted with permission from the Society of Thoracic Surgeons.)

rejection in infants and children is formed from clinical evidence, echocardiography, and endomyocardial biopsy. Although some centers have relied heavily on routine endomyocardial biopsy for the diagnosis of acute rejection with a similar frequency to that used in adults, this has the disadvantage of requiring general anesthesia and potentially the loss of venous access. Clinical clues to the presence of acute cardiac rejection include alterations in the child's activity level, listlessness, poor feeding, atrial and ventricular ectopy, persisting resting tachycardia, and evidence of heart failure. Others have placed a great deal of reliance on the echocardiographic detection of acute cardiac rejection. A number of echocardiographic changes that reflect an increase in left ventricular mass and impairment of systolic and diastolic function (reduction of left ventricular posterior thickening fraction, left ventricular shortening fraction, and left ventricular posterior wall thinning velocity) have been reported to correlate with histologic evidence of acute cardiac rejection.[32–34] Regardless of which method of detection is predominantly used, it would seem prudent to incorporate all three modalities into a strategy of surveillance for acute cardiac rejection.

Treatment of acute cardiac rejection, as in adult cardiac transplantation, is based on the histologic grade of rejection and its hemodynamic effects. Treatment includes pulse steroid therapy, antilymphocyte globulin, and OKT3 therapy. Other modalities have been used to treat persistent and recalcitrant rejection, including methotrexate[35, 36] and total lymphoid irradiation.[37]

INFECTION

The incidence of infection and infection-related death is highest the first few months after transplantation, reflecting a period of heightened immunosuppression and the increased risk of infection associated with the postoperative period.[38] As in adults, cytomegalovirus infection is particularly problematic. The highest risk of a serious primary infection occurs in seronegative patients who have received a heart from a seropositive donor or have received a blood transfusion with cytomegalovirus-positive blood. Respiratory tract infection with respiratory syncytial virus[39] is particularly common in children younger than 6 months, with the potential long-term sequelae of significant reactive airway disease.[40]

CORONARY ALLOGRAFT VASCULOPATHY

Coronary allograft vasculopathy is a major long-term limiting factor to survival after cardiac transplantation. Its pathogenesis involves a complex interaction between traditional atherogenic factors and transplant-related factors such as frequency of acute cardiac rejection and prior cytomegalovirus infection. Coronary allograft vasculopathy in adults is detected in more than 80% of long-term survivors by 8 years after cardiac transplantation, is progressive,[41] and the traditional method of detection by coronary angiography importantly underestimates the incidence and severity of the disease.[42, 43] The pathologic features are identical in infants and children to those in adults.[44] A study by Pahl et al. which involved a multicenter national survey, concluded that the incidence of coronary allograft vasculopathy in children is similar to that in adult transplant recipients.[45] As in adult patients, a significant number of children died late after cardiac transplantation of coronary allograft vasculopathy despite having a recent normal coronary angiogram. These investigators also found a relationship between increased frequency of acute cellular rejection and the subsequent development of coronary allograft vasculopathy. The challenge of the future to minimize the incidence and consequences of this serious problem is to decrease the immunologic insult to the endothelium, improve detection (perhaps intracoronary US), and develop strategies for treatment and prevention by modification of traditional atherogenic risk factors.

SURVIVAL

In a study by Shaddy and colleagues from the Pediatric Heart Transplant Study, the survival of children after cardiac transplantation

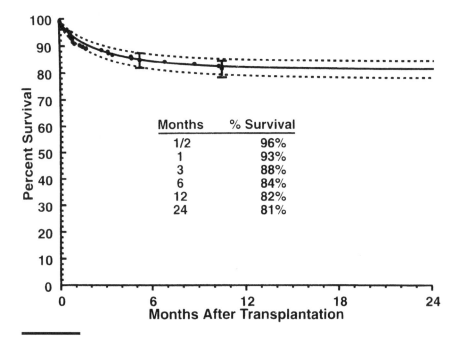

Months	% Survival
1/2	96%
1	93%
3	88%
6	84%
12	82%
24	81%

FIGURE 13.

Patient survival in 191 pediatric patients between the ages of 1 and 18 years undergoing heart transplantation between January 1993 and December 1994 at PHTS centers. *Dashed lines* enclose the 70% confidence limits. (Courtesy of Shaddy RE, Naftel DC, Kirklin JK, et al: Outcome of cardiac transplantation in children: Survival in a contemporary multi-institutional experience. *Circulation* 94:69–73. Copyright 1996, American Heart Association. Reproduced with permission.)

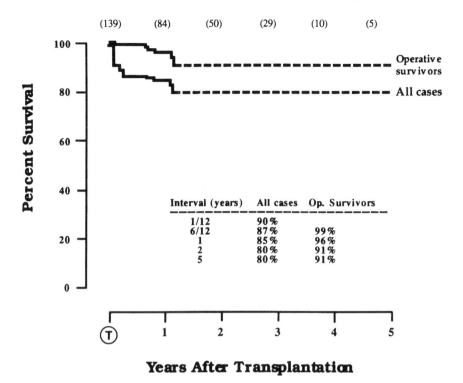

FIGURE 14.

Survival curve (Kaplan-Meier estimate) after heart transplantation in first year of life. *Bottom line* shows survival of the 139 infants. *Top line* shows operative survivors. The *numbers in parentheses* represent patients at risk beyond that time. *Horizontal dashed lines* show event-free patients. (Courtesy of Bailey LL, Gundry SR, Razzouk AJ, et al: Bless the babies: One hundred fifteen late survivors of heart transplantation during the first year of life. *J Thorac Cardiovasc Surg* 105:805–815, 1993.)

in a contemporary multi-institutional experience was examined.[15] Survival at 2 years after cardiac transplantation was 81% (Fig 13). By multivariable analysis, the presence of a ventricular assist device and/or intra-aortic balloon pump at the time of transplantation was identified as a risk factor for death ($P = 0.02$). The survival of patients with these devices was significantly reduced, with a 2-month survival of 70% compared with 92% in patients without a device. In this study, 31 of 191 patients who underwent cardiac transplantation died. The major causes of death were rejection (29% of deaths), early graft failure (19%), infection (16%), sudden death (13%), and other causes (23%). The survival of infants after cardiac transplantation in the first year of life at Loma Linda[4] demonstrates the remarkable progress that has been made. Actuarial survival of these patients (Fig 14) is 80% five years after transplantation. Survival of the 60 neonates who had cardiac transplantation at Loma Linda was 84% at 5 years.[4]

CARDIAC GROWTH AFTER TRANSPLANTATION

Increasing evidence suggests that after cardiac transplantation in infants and children, the heart undergoes relatively normal growth in terms of left ventricular volume and muscle mass in proportion to the body's surface area (Fig 15).[46] Furthermore, left ventricular ejection fraction and cardiac index remain normal, although there is evidence of restrictive physiology.[47]

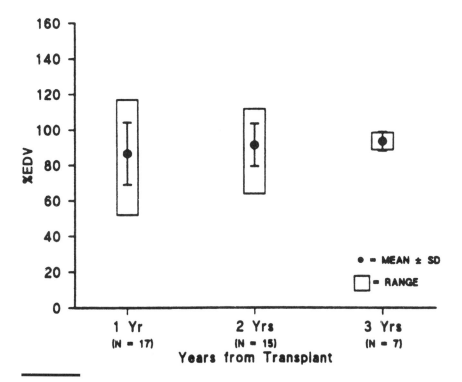

FIGURE 15.
Plot of values for left ventricular end-diastolic volume predicted for body surface area demonstrating adaptation of donor heart volume to recipient body size. *Abbreviation: %EDV*, left ventricular end-diastolic volume predicted for body surface area. (Courtesy of Zales VR, Wright KL, Muster AJ, et al: ventricular volume growth after cardiac transplantation in infants and children. *Circulation* 86:272–275. Copyright 1992, American Heart Association. Reproduced with permission.)

SOMATIC GROWTH AND DEVELOPMENT

As demonstrated by a study by Baum and colleagues,[48] the majority of infants undergoing cardiac transplantation experience relatively normal growth. Infants who underwent late transplantation (mean, 68 days after birth) compared with those undergoing early transplantation (mean, 18 days after birth) were smaller, but these differences were no longer apparent 6 months after transplantation. The developmental outcome for the majority of patients after cardiac transplantation was within the normal range, although a few did have evidence of important neurologic handicaps.[48] Four months after cardiac transplantation, 19% of infants had an abnormal neurologic examination, with the most common finding being generalized hypotonia.

FUTURE PROGRESS

Considerable progress has been made in the science and practice of pediatric cardiac transplantation, but many unresolved issues persist. Increasing the number of donor hearts is a pressing issue, and the solution to this problem may lie with xenotransplantation and the use of anencephalic donors, as well as other novel strategies such as the use of hearts after resuscitation of asystolic donors. Improvements in immunosuppression and strategies to induce tolerance would significantly enhance long-term survival. When the results of pediatric cardiac transplantation become more predictable and the procedure becomes more generally applicable, the true role of this therapy in the management of complex congenital heart disease for which other therapies are currently available can be better defined.

REFERENCES

1. Kantrowitz A, Haller JD, Joos H, et al: Transplantation of the heart in an infant and an adult. *Am J Cardiol* 22:782–790, 1968.
2. Cooley DA, Bloodwell RD, Hallman GL, et al: Organ transplantation for advanced cardiopulmonary disease. *Ann Thorac Surg* 8:30–46, 1969.
3. Yacoub MH, Radley-Smith R: Heart transplantation in infants and children. *Semin Thorac Cardiovasc Surg* 2:206–212, 1990.
4. Bailey LL, Gundry SR, Razzouk AJ, et al: Bless the babies: One hundred fifteen late survivors of heart transplantation during the first year of life. *J Thorac Cardiovasc Surg* 105:805–815, 1993.
5. Bailey LL, Nehlsen-Cannarella SL, Concepcion W, et al: Baboon-to-human cardiac xenotransplantation in a neonate. *JAMA* 254:3321–3329, 1985.
6. Report of the WHO/ISFC task force on definition and classification of cardiomyopathies. *Br Heart J* 44:672–673, 1980.

7. Chen SC, Nouri S, Balfour I, et al: Clinical profile of congestive cardiomyopathy in children. *J Am Coll Cardiol* 15:189–193, 1990.

8. Matitiau A, Perez-Atayde A, Sanders SP, et al: Infantile dilated cardiomyopathy: Relation of outcome to left ventricular mechanics, hemodynamics, and histology at the time of presentation. *Circulation* 90:1310–1318, 1994.

9. Talierico CP, Seward JB, Driscoll DJ, et al: Idiopathic dilated cardiomyopathy in the young: Clinical profile and natural history. *J Am Coll Cardiol* 6:1126–1131, 1985.

10. Griffin ML, Hernandez A, Martin TC, et al: Dilated cardiomyopathy in infants and children. *J Am Coll Cardiol* 11:139–144, 1988.

11. Friedman RA, Moak JP, Garson A: Clinical course of idiopathic dilated cardiomyopathy in children. *J Am Coll Cardiol* 18:152–156, 1991.

12. Drucker NA, Colan SD, Lewis AB, et al: Gamma globulin treatment of acute myocarditis in the pediatric population. *Circulation* 89:252–257, 1994.

13. Wigle ED, Rakowski H, Kimball BP, et al: Hypertrophic cardiomyopathy: Clinical spectrum and treatment. *Circulation* 92:1680–1692, 1995.

14. Lewis AB: Clinical profile and outcome of restrictive cardiomyopathy in children. *Am Heart J* 123:1589–1593, 1992.

15. Shaddy RE, Naftel DC, Kirklin JK, et al: Outcome of cardiac transplantation in children: Survival in a contemporary multi-institutional experience. *Circulation* 94:69–73, 1996.

16. Kinsella JP, Neish SR, Shaffer E, et al: Low-dose inhalational nitric oxide in persistent pulmonary hypertension of the newborn. *Lancet* 340:819–820, 1992.

17. Kaplan EL, Meier P: Nonparametric estimation from incomplete observations. *J Am Stat Assoc* 53:457–481, 1958.

18. McGiffin DC, Naftel DC, Kirklin JK, et al: Predicting outcome following listing for cardiac transplantation in children: Comparison of Kaplan-Meier and parametric competing risk analysis. *J Heart Lung Transplant,* in press.

19. President's Commission for the Study of Ethical Problems in Medicine and Biomedical and Behavioral Research: Guidelines for the determination of death. Special communication. *JAMA* 246:2184–2186, 1981.

20. Ashwal S, Caplan AL, Cheatham WA, et al: Session IX: Social and ethical controversies in pediatric heart transplantation. *J Heart Lung Transplant* 10:860–876, 1991.

21. Backer CL, Zales VR, Idriss FS, et al: Heart transplantation in neonates and in children. *J Heart Lung Transplant* 11:311–319, 1992.

22. Boucek MM, Mathis CM, Kanakriyeh MS, et al: Donor shortage: Use of the dysfunctional donor heart. *J Heart Lung Transplant* 12:186S–S190S, 1993.

23. Kawauchi M, Gundry SR, de Begona JA, et al: Utilization of pediatric donors salvaged by cardiopulmonary resuscitation. *J Heart Lung Transplant* 12:185–188, 1993.

24. Fullerton DA, Gundry SR, de Begona JA, et al: The effects of donor-recipient size disparity in infant and pediatric heart transplantation. *J Thorac Cardiovasc Surg* 104:1314–1419, 1992.
25. Tamisier D, Vouhe P, Le Bidois J, et al: Donor-recipient size matching in pediatric heart transplantation: A word of caution about small grafts. *J Heart Lung Transplant* 15:190–195, 1996.
26. Kawauchi M, Gundry SR, Beierle F, et al: Myosin light chain efflux after heart transplantation in infants and children and its correlation with ischemic preservation time. *J Thorac Cardiovasc Surg* 106:458–462, 1993.
27. Bailey LL: Heart transplantation techniques in complex congenital heart disease. *J Heart Lung Transplant* 12:168S–175S, 1993.
28. Bailey L, Concepcion W, Shattuck H, et al: Method of heart transplantation for treatment of hypoplastic left heart syndrome. *J Thorac Cardiovasc Surg* 92:1, 1986.
29. Backer CL, Idriss FS, Zales VR, et al: Cardiac transplantation for hypoplastic left heart syndrome: A modified technique. *Ann Thorac Surg* 50:894–898, 1990.
30. Bailey L, Kahan B, Nehlsen-Cannarella S, et al: Session V: The neonatal immune system: Window of opportunity? *J Heart Lung Transplant* 10:828–829, 1991.
31. Canter CE, Moorhead S, Saffitz JE, et al: Steroid withdrawal in the pediatric heart transplant recipient initially treated with triple immunosuppression. *J Heart Lung Transplant* 13:74–80, 1994.
32. Boucek MM, Mathis CM, Boucek RJ, et al: Prospective evaluation of echocardiography for primary rejection surveillance after infant heart transplantation: Comparison with endomyocardial biopsy. *J Heart Lung Transplant* 13:66–73, 1994.
33. Tantengco MV, Dodd D, Frist WH, et al: Echocardiographic abnormalities with acute cardiac allograft rejection in children: Correlation with endomyocardial biopsy. *J Heart Lung Transplant* 12:203S–210S, 1993.
34. Loker J, Darragh R, Ensing G, et al: Echocardiographic analysis of rejection in the infant heart transplant recipient. *J Heart Lung Transplant* 13:1014–1018, 1994.
35. Bouchart F, Gundry SR, Schaack-Gonzales JV, et al: Methotrexate as rescue/adjunctive immunotherapy in infant and adult heart transplantation. *J Heart Lung Transplant* 12:427–433, 1993.
36. Shaddy RE, Bullock EA, Tani LY, et al: Methotrexate therapy in pediatric heart transplantation as treatment of recurrent mild to moderate acute cellular rejection. *J Heart Lung Transplant* 13:1009–1013, 1994.
37. Bernstein D, Miller J, Reitz B, et al: Total lymphoid irradiation (TLI) for treatment of intractable rejection in pediatric heart transplant recipients. *J Heart Lung Transplant* 13:42A, 1994.
38. Sarris GE, Smith JA, Bernstein D, et al: Pediatric cardiac transplantation: The Stanford experience. *Circulation* 90:51–55, 1994.
39. Bork J, Chinnock R, Ogata K, et al: Infectious complications in infant heart transplantation. *J Heart Lung Transplant* 12:199S–202S, 1993.

40. Bork JM, Baum M, Rincon D, et al: Acute respiratory syncytial virus infection in infant heart transplant patients (abstract). Presented at the meeting of the Western Society for Pediatric Research, Carmel, Calif, February 1991.

41. McGiffin DC, Savunen T, Kirklin JK, et al: Cardiac transplant coronary artery disease: A multivariable analysis of pretransplantation risk factors for disease development and morbid events. *J Thorac Cardiovasc Surg* 109:1081–1089, 1995.

42. Johnson DE, Alderman EL, Schroeder JS, et al: Transplant coronary artery disease: Histopathologic correlations with angiographic morphology. *J Am Coll Cardiol* 17:449–457, 1991.

43. O'Neill BJ, Pflugfelder PW, Singh NR, et al: Frequency of angiographic detection and quantitative assessment of coronary arterial disease one and three years after cardiac transplantation. *Am J Cardiol* 63:1221–1226, 1989.

44. Berry GJ, Rizeq MN, Weiss LM, et al: Graft coronary disease in pediatric heart and combined heart-lung transplant recipients: A study of fifteen cases. *J Heart Lung Transplant* 12:309S–319S, 1993.

45. Pahl E, Zales VR, Fricker FJ, et al: Posttransplant coronary artery disease in children: A multicenter national survey. *Circulation* 90:56–60, 1994.

46. Zales VR, Wright KL, Muster AJ, et al: Ventricular volume growth after cardiac transplantation in infants and children. *Circulation* 86:272–275, 1992.

47. Zales VR, Wright KL, Pahl E, et al: Normal left ventricular muscle mass and mass/volume ratio after pediatric cardiac transplantation. *Circulation* 90:61–65, 1994.

48. Baum M, Chinnock R, Ashwal S, et al: Growth and neurodevelopmental outcome of infants undergoing heart transplantation. *J Heart Lung Transplant* 12:211S–217S, 1993.

CHAPTER 10

Surgery for Kawasaki Disease

Soichiro Kitamura, M.D.
Professor of Surgery, Department of Surgery III, Nara Medical College, Kashihara Nara, Japan

Yoichi Kameda, M.D.
Research Associate of Surgery, Department of Surgery III, Nara Medical College, Kashihara Nara, Japan

Yasunaru Kawashima, M.D.
President Emenitus, National Cardiovascular Center, Suita, Osaka, Japan

K awasaki disease (KD), first reported by Kawasaki and colleagues in 1967,[1, 2] has now been diagnosed widely throughout the world,[3] with a particularly high incidence in Japan. Its etiologic pathogen, along with the basic mechanism of immune allergy causing angiitis, has yet to be clarified. Valvular lesions, myocarditis, arrhythmias, and pericarditis are all recognized as sequelae within the heart, in addition to ischemic heart disease caused by obstructive lesions of the coronary arteries. Aortic and peripheral aneurysms are also reported as sequelae of systemic arteritis. Serious coronary arterial disease and valvular disease resistant to medical treatment are the major indications for surgical treatment.[4–6] Coronary arterial disease, in particular, has a high incidence and causes serious myocardial dysfunction and sudden death.[7, 8] Recent progress in γ-globulin therapy[9, 10] for acute KD has decreased coronary artery complications, but the lesions continue to occur. This has, therefore, been an area for which suitable treatment is most urgently sought. Surgical myocardial revascularization has shown efficacy specifically for inflammatory coronary artery aneurysms and obstruction.[11]

ISCHEMIC HEART DISEASE IN CHILDREN WITH KAWASAKI DISEASE: LESIONS OF THE CORONARY ARTERIES

During the acute stage of KD, before the use of IV γ-globulin, dilatation of the coronary arteries occurred in approximately 50% of the

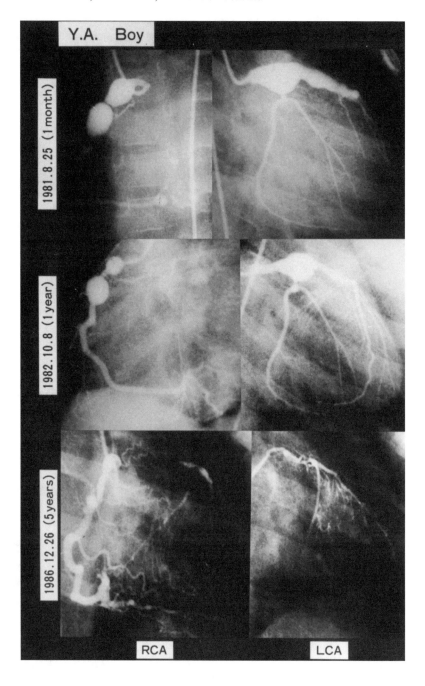

patients, 10% to 20% of whom were found to have coronary arterial aneurysms after subsidence of the acute febrile symptoms.[12] Rupture of aneurysms and coronary thrombosis were the leading causes of death during the acute illness,[13] but surgical interventions have rarely been performed except for relief of acute cardiac tamponade. Even if aneurysms develop at the acute stage, more than half of the patients show regression, with normal angiograms detected during the course of 1–2 years.[14, 15] Fewer than half of the afflicted patients retain aneurysms or irregular lumina of the coronary arteries, and stenotic and occlusive lesions resulting in ischemic heart disease occur in only 3% of these children. Coronary angiograms depicting progression to coronary obstruction are shown in Figure 1. The recent use of γ-globulin at the acute stage has reduced the incidence of coronary dilatation to 15%, but coronary involvement still continues to occur. An arterial aneurysm of large size but not associated with a stenotic lesion has been demonstrated to hydrodynamically produce a stenotic effect.[16] Such lesions, however, rarely cause clinically evident myocardial ischemia. As far as the authors know, there has as yet been no report of rupture of an aneurysm in long-term follow-up after convalescence from the acute disease because of the resulting thick and hard arterial wall healing from acute inflammation. The indication for surgery is, therefore, not established by the mere presence of coronary arterial aneurysms. Children with large aneurysms (8 mm in diameter or greater) or multiple aneurysms, nonetheless, have a high incidence of later stenosis and obstruction at the entrance and exit of the aneurysm, which results in myocardial infarction. Thus surgical treatment is generally reserved for children with large or multiple aneurysms and resultant occlusive changes.

Kato et al.,[17] reporting on behalf of a group working for the Japanese Ministry of Health and Welfare, found that 43 children (22%) died out of 195 having an initial myocardial infarction. Among these, the incidence of so-called sudden death was noted

---

FIGURE 1.
Progression of coronary obstructive disease from the coronary aneurysms in Kawasaki disease. Large right and left coronary artery *(RCA and LCA)* aneurysms formed at the age of 1 month **(upper panels).** Some regression of the aneurysms was observed 1 year after the onset of disease **(middle panels),** but severe obstructive lesions developed 5 years after the disease **(bottom panels).** (Courtesy of Kitamura S: Surgical management for cardiovascular lesions in Kawasaki disease. *Cardiol Young* 1:240–253, 1991.)

to be 61%. Of the surviving 152 children, 24 (16%) had a recurrence of myocardial infarction and 15 (63%) died. Six of the remaining 9 children had a third recurrence of myocardial infarction, with 5 (83%) of these patients dying. The mortality of myocardial infarction in children is thus not low by any means and demonstrates the need for surgical treatment in a group of patients who may otherwise die.

SYMPTOMS, DIAGNOSIS, AND INDICATIONS FOR SURGICAL TREATMENT

When an occlusive lesion is found in one or more major coronary arteries and the large area of cardiac muscle supplied by the artery is ischemic but viable, myocardial revascularization is indicated, usually by surgical means and occasionally by percutaneous transluminal coronary angioplasty or directional coronary atherectomy.[18] In this situation, the subjects are children, and despite the presence of serious coronary arterial involvement, subjective symptoms of myocardial ischemia may be poorly expressed and the occurrence of death is usually sudden.[8, 17] Objective findings from various examinations are therefore important for determining the need for surgical treatment. The standard indication for surgical treatment has been discussed in the study group of the Japanese Ministry of Health and Welfare and reported elsewhere.[6, 11] The specific ischemic region and the viability of myocardium should be determined by exercise ECG with the treadmill test and/or myocardial imaging with thallium-201 under exercise or the administration of drugs such as dipyridamole, in addition to clinical findings, including a history of angina pectoris and myocardial infarction. Even though the subjects are children, left ventriculography and selective coronary angiography are essential for determining the indication for surgery. Indications for surgery should be determined with care and take into consideration patient age, history of myocardial infarction, and left ventricular function, in addition to the coronary arteriography findings.[6, 19]

The indications resemble those for coronary artery bypass surgery in adults. In KD, however, several characteristics specific to children are found in the angiographic findings. First, when one of the major coronary arteries is occluded, the ability to form collateral vessels in children is very high, probably because of increased blood levels of various growth factors. Left ventricular wall motion is moderately reduced in many cases, perhaps secondary to coexistent myocarditis at the acute stage of this disease.[7]

Second, recanalization of the coronary artery is frequently noted at the point of occlusion, particularly in the right coronary artery. When lesions are limited to the right coronary artery, patients are often asymptomatic, but lesions frequently coexist in the left coronary artery.[20] Thus when ischemia is identified by various tests, surgery is indicated. Surgical treatment is also recommended when myocardial infarction has previously occurred because of the high incidence of infarct recurrence.[17]

SURGICAL TREATMENT

Surgical myocardial revascularization has been increasingly performed for this disease since 1976, when we reported the first successful coronary artery bypass operation using grafts prepared from the saphenous vein.[21] Since then, several questions relating to surgical treatment have been resolved. First, coronary arterial bypass surgery is safe and effective for inflammatory coronary artery disease secondary to KD in children. Second, the main locations of coronary arterial obstruction in KD are fortunately in the proximal portions of major coronary arteries. Thus if the caliber of the coronary arteries is not too small in infants, the operation can be performed anywhere in the coronary arterial system. Coronary artery stenosis or obstruction caused by KD in 168 surgical patients enrolled in a multicenter cooperative study[22] is shown in Figure 2. The third consideration, which is one of the most important issues in surgical treatment, is that long-term patency of the autologous saphenous vein graft in children undergoing surgery at a younger age is unsatisfactory. Fourth, it has been shown that an internal thoracic artery (ITA) graft can be successfully used in children with a similar favorable patency as that found in adults.[23, 24]

Surgical revascularization for KD has developed and progressed mainly in Japan, where the incidence of the disease is high. Reports of operations performed in various other countries are now increasingly available.[25–29] The indications for surgery and the modes of treatment have now been fairly well established, with satisfactory results; however, some issues remain regarding the long-term results of coronary artery bypass surgery in children beyond 10 years and after their growth into adulthood.[30] The effect of older age, when atherosclerosis more commonly occurs, is expected to affect the long-term outcome. Intimal injuries secondary to Kawasaki angiitis may become fertile soil for atherosclerotic changes.[13, 31]

MODES OF TREATMENT

CORONARY ARTERY BYPASS GRAFTING

Because coronary artery lesions usually occur in the proximal portions of the coronary arteries in patients with KD, bypass grafting

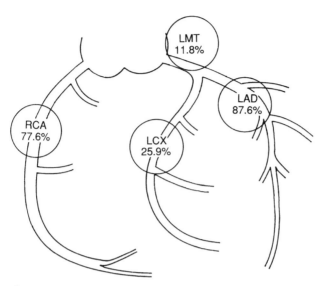

Coronary Artery Stenosis and Obstructions

FIGURE 2.

Coronary artery stenosis or obstruction caused by Kawasaki disease in 168 surgical patients enrolled in a multicenter cooperative study.[22] Obstructive disease developed at the inflow or outflow sites of the coronary aneurysms, generally located in the proximal portion of the coronary artery. The left anterior descending *(LAD)* artery was most commonly involved, followed by the right coronary artery *(RCA)*, left circumflex *(LCX)* artery, and the left main trunk *(LMT)* in that order. (Courtesy of Kitamura S, Kameda Y, Seki T, et al: Long-term outcome of myocardial revascularization in patients with Kawasaki coronary artery disease. *J Thorac Cardiovasc Surg* 107:663–674, 1994.)

is applicable in most patients, even at the age of 1 or 2, unless the coronary arteries are too small. In terms of the nature of the graft, autologous saphenous veins,[4, 16, 21, 25, 26] the ITA, or a combination of both grafts is usually used. Since our report[23, 24] showing favorable long-term patency results of a graft constructed from the ITA, this technique has been used with increasing frequency.[24, 27, 29, 32] The use of bilateral ITAs is also recommended because this practice does not adversely affect development of the chest wall in children.[33] The gastroepiploic artery has also been used with early favorable result.[34–36] All efforts to use in situ arterial grafts are based on the unsatisfactory long-term patency of autologous saphenous veins in the pediatric population. In children, both the ITA and the coronary arteries are small. It is therefore advisable to use microsurgical techniques when anastomosing vessels 1 mm in diameter, ideally with the help of a surgical microscope or high-power magnifying loupes (over 3× to 10× magnification). Representative postoperative angiograms are shown in Figures 3 and 4; bilateral ITA grafts or left ITA and gastroepiploic artery grafts were used to revascularize a coronary artery obstructed because of KD.

CORONARY ANEURYSMECTOMY

The combined use of coronary artery bypass grating with resection of large coronary aneurysms has been reported.[16] Coronary aneurysms caused by this disease are not reported to rupture except at the acute febrile stage, probably because of extensive fibrosis and thickening around the aneurysm as a result of healing of severe inflammation in the vessel wall. This is different from aneurysms caused by atherosclerosis. Thus aneurysmectomy is rarely recommended as a mode of surgical treatment for the sequelae of KD.

OPTIMAL AGE FOR SURGERY

Because the long-term patency of grafts prepared from saphenous veins is unsatisfactory, particularly in patients who underwent

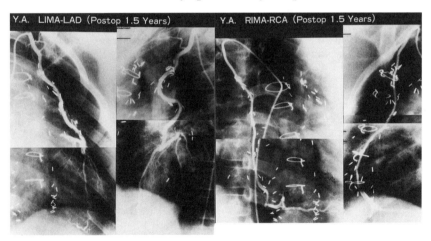

FIGURE 3.

Same patient as in Figure 1. This child underwent bilateral internal thoracic (mammary) artery (ITA) grafting, and postoperative angiograms demonstrated an enlarged left ITA graft to the left anterior descending *(LAD)* artery, as well as a widely patent right ITA graft to the right coronary artery *(RCA)*. This boy plays on the soccer team at school with no restrictions. *Abbreviations: LIMA,* left internal mammary artery; *RIMA,* right internal mammary artery. (Courtesy of Kitamura S, Kawachi K, Seki T, et al: Bilateral internal mammary artery grafts for coronary bypass operations in children. *J Thorac Cardiovasc Surg* 99:708–715, 1990.)

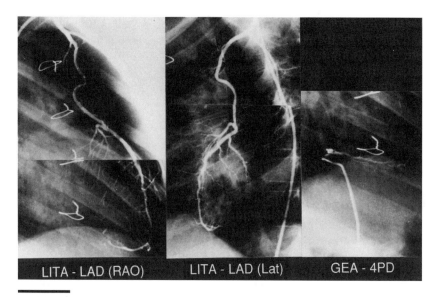

FIGURE 4.

Use of an internal thoracic artery graft and the gastroepiploic artery *(GEA)* to revascularize the left anterior descending *(LAD)* artery and the posterior descending artery in a 5-year-old boy with total occlusion of the LAD and the recanalized right coronary artery. *Abbreviations: LITA,* left internal thoracic artery; *RAO,* right anterior oblique; *Lat,* lateral; *4PD,* posterior descending artery.

coronary artery bypass operations at a younger age, indications for surgery should be determined with care. In younger children (less than 2 years old), it is sometimes better to delay surgery under strict medical control and monitor with appropriately repeated coronary arteriography because the age at surgery is a significant risk factor for hospital and late death.[22] In serious cases, however, surgery should be performed regardless of the child's age. For very young children, the ITA should be used as the graft of choice because of its expected growth in length and caliber and excellent long-term patency.[24] Whenever necessary and feasible, we recommend the utilization of bilateral ITA grafts. Harvesting both ITAs does not harm chest wall growth.[33] Serious obstructive lesions and symptoms are rare in very young children, however, and occlusive lesions usually develop at least several years and usually more than 10 years after the onset of KD. In children older than the age of 5 years, less difficulty is expected in surgical procedures because of the size of the coronary arteries. Accordingly, it may be desirable to manage patients with intensive medical management and observation. The youngest patient in one of the author's series (S.K.) is a child of 1 year and the oldest is 19 years, the mean age being 9.6 ± 4.3 years (n = 51). The majority of patients were 5–6 years of age.

SURGICAL RESULTS
SURVIVAL RATES
The results of coronary artery bypass grafting in children with KD are now quite good. According to investigations conducted by the multicenter cooperative group,[22] only 2 patients died in the hospital among 170 undergoing surgery for KD. In this study, 8 patients (4.7%) died suddenly or as a result of myocardial infarction in the 90-month period follow-up after surgery. Causes of death included left ventricular dysfunction, arrhythmia, and late occlusion of grafts. Of note, the lack of an ITA graft (particularly to the left anterior descending artery) is a strong predictor of late postoperative death.[22]

SURGICAL EFFECTS AND POSTOPERATIVE CARDIAC EVENTS
Coronary artery bypass surgery for patients with KD is useful for improving angina pectoris. This is objectively demonstrated by exercise ECG and myocardial perfusion imaging, both of which show evidence of increased myocardial perfusion after surgery.[32, 34] Postoperative improvement in blood flow measured in the coronary sinus and improvement in left ventricular function under exercise loading have also been noted.[37] Before surgery, most children were totally restricted from the physical exercise program at school, but after surgery, the rate of return to normal school athletics was as high as 70%.[20] Bypass surgery is effective in improving the quality of life of children with severe coronary sequelae of KD. In a multicenter cooperative study[22] including 168 postoperative patients, 84% of the patients were in good health after the operation, and there were no postoperative cardiac events in 71.4% of the patients. Mild ischemia was detected after the operation in 14.3% of the patients either by stress ECG or by thallium scintigraphy, and clinical angina pectoris persisted or recurred in 6.5% of the patients. Myocardial infarction recurred in 2.4%, and severe ventricular arrhythmias were seen in 1.2% of the patients. Postoperative ischemic events were relatively prevalent, totaling 24.4% in the multicenter study.[22] Causes of these events included incomplete revascularization at the time of surgery, mostly because of technical difficulty in small children; high graft occlusion rates, progression of coronary dilatation to obstruction late after the operation; and possible coexisting sequelae of myocarditis.[38, 39]

PATENCY OF GRAFTS

The efficacy of coronary artery bypass surgery largely depends on long-term patency of the grafts. Patency of the previously used autologous saphenous vein is not satisfactory (Fig 5). The venous graft used in children, particularly younger children, has been found to have a high occlusion rate. The patency rate of venous grafts has been compared in children younger than 7 years and older than 7 years of age. The early patency rate was 65.4% ± 7.9% 84 months after the operation in those 8 years of age and older vs. 27.7% ± 8.1% (*P* < 0.01) in those younger than 7 years[22] (Fig 6). In addition, occlusion was noted more frequently in follow-ups beyond 1 year. This finding appears to be unrelated to technical factors alone. The rate of degeneration of venous grafts is possibly higher in younger children. In childhood, metabolism related to growth differs from that in adults. For instance, xenograft valves implanted

Graft Patency Rates

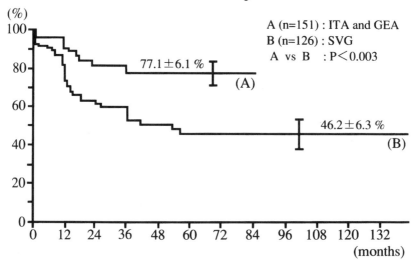

FIGURE 5.

Comparison of actuarial overall graft patency rates between arterial grafts *(A)* (*n* = 151) and venous grafts *(B)* (*n* = 126). Arterial grafts demonstrated a significantly higher angiographic patency rate than did venous grafts. Occlusion of venous grafts was common during the first few years after surgery. *Abbreviations: ITA,* internal thoracic artery; *GEA,* gastroepiploic artery; *SVG,* saphenous vein graft. (Courtesy of Kitamura S, Kameda Y, Seki T, et al: Long-term outcome of myocardial revascularization in patients with Kawasaki coronary artery disease. *J Thorac Cardiovasc Surg* 107:663–674, 1994.)

Graft Patency Rates in Patients under 7 Years of Age

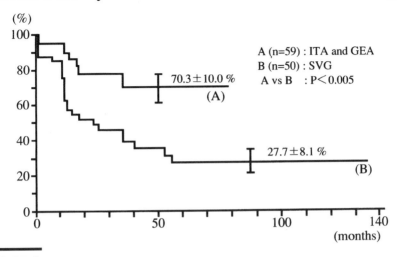

FIGURE 6.

Comparison of actuarial graft patency rates between arterial grafts *(A) (n* = 59) and venous grafts *(B) (n* = 50) in children less than 7 years of age at surgery. The saphenous vein graft *(SVG)* patency rate was remarkably low. *Abbreviations: ITA,* internal thoracic artery; *GEA,* gastroepiploic artery. (Courtesy of Kitamura S, Kameda Y, Seki T, et al: Long-term outcome of myocardial revascularization in patients with Kawasaki coronary artery disease. *J Thorac Cardiovasc Surg* 107:663–674, 1994.)

in childhood become readily calcified and fail to function in a few years. It has now been demonstrated that the saphenous vein, although autologous in origin when used as a free graft, has no potential to grow longitudinally in a fashion corresponding to the somatic growth of the patients.[24] When providing myocardial revascularization for sequelae of KD, the saphenous vein is not an appropriate graft, particularly in children aged less than 7 years. We believe that the use of vein grafts for pediatric myocardial revascularization should be avoided if at all possible.

Use of the ITA was anticipated to overcome the disadvantages of the vein graft. The arterial graft has been shown to have excellent long-term patency in adults, but its use in children seemed at first difficult because of the small caliber of the blood vessels. After our successful report of the use of an arterial graft in children with KD,[23] however, more operations have been performed with this technique.* When the rate of patency of venous grafts was

*References 23, 24, 27, 29, 32, 33, 36.

compared with that of arterial grafts in one of the author's series (S.K.) ($n = 51$), the patency rate was 95% for the arterial and 91% for the venous graft within 1 month after surgery, but this difference was not statistically significant. The patency rate of the venous graft after a period of follow-up longer than 1 year after surgery, however, decreased to 49% at 10 years, whereas arterial grafts maintained a patency rate of 89.5% at 10 years. The patency rate of the arterial graft is therefore significantly ($P = 0.0002$) better. This is confirmed by the multicenter study,[22] which included a larger number of grafts. Arterial grafts (ITA and gastroepiploic artery, $n = 151$) showed a significantly higher angiographic patency rate than did venous grafts ($n = 126$): 77.1% $\pm$ 6.1% vs. 46.2% $\pm$ 6.3%, $P < 0.003$ (see Fig 5). Although the numbers are small, patency of the gastroepiploic artery also seemed to be promising in our experience, as well as that of others.[34–36]

GROWTH POTENTIAL OF ARTERIAL GRAFTS

When the length of ITA grafts early after surgery was compared with the length at late follow-up, longitudinal growth consistent with growth of the child was demonstrated.[24] A close correlation was found between the length of the arterial graft and the increase in body surface area or body height of the patient, as illustrated in Figures 7 and 8. The method of measuring ITA graft length within the chest has been detailed elsewhere.[24]

In addition, the diameter of the ITA as well as the anastomosis can increase significantly in accordance with the flow requirement and growth of the patient.[24, 33, 34] Thus the ITA is a very suitable graft for pediatric patients not only with KD but also with congenital coronary anomalies who require coronary artery bypass surgery.[40, 41] Because there are only two ITAs, the gastroepiploic artery has also begun to be used in pediatric coronary artery bypass surgery. We have used this artery in 8 of 51 patients with promising results.

VALVULAR DISEASE SECONDARY TO KAWASAKI DISEASE

MITRAL REGURGITATION

In KD, mitral regurgitation is occasionally produced as a result of dysfunction of the papillary muscle. This dysfunction may be caused by myocarditis, valvulitis, or ischemia secondary to coronary artery involvement. Mild regurgitation may also be observed during the acute febrile period of the disease, which regresses spontaneously in most instances. In patients with advanced regurgitation lasting throughout the period of convalescence and serious enough to cause cardiac failure, surgical treatment should be considered.[5, 23] Pathologic findings of the mitral valvular apparatus in patients with regurgitation secondary to KD include ruptured chordae tendineae,[42] fibrous nodules within the valvular leaflets, and necrosis, fibrosis, and atrophy of myocardial cells in the papillary muscles.[5, 20]

When determining indications for surgery, it is important to consider the degree of regurgitation, age of the patient, lesions of the coronary arteries, and left ventricular function. Mitral regurgitation in patients with KD is different from that seen in those with

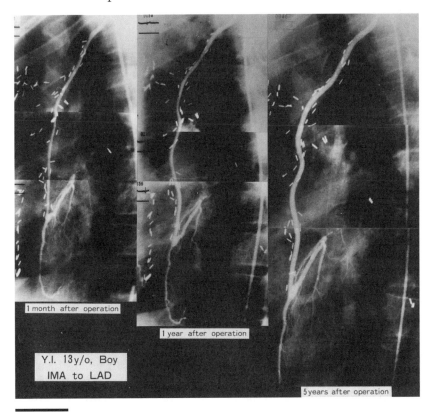

FIGURE 7.

Chronological changes occurring in an internal thoracic (mammary) artery graft anastomosed to the left anterior descending *(LAD)* artery. Three angiograms were taken at different periods after surgery (1 month, 1 year, and 5 years) with nearly equal magnification (see the size of the clips—3.5 mm in length). Longitudinal as well as circumferential development in line with somatic growth of the patient is apparent. *Abbreviation: IMA,* internal mammary artery.

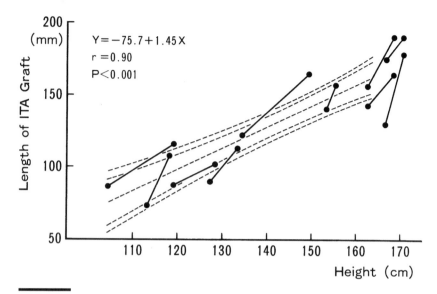

FIGURE 8.

Relationship between the increase in length of internal thoracic artery *(ITA)* grafts and the increase in patient height. A significant correlation is apparent and reveals biological viability of the graft in response to somatic growth.

rheumatic valvular disease because, first, complicating coronary artery lesions are frequently associated and require simultaneous surgery and, second, significantly depressed left ventricular function is noted in many patients.[5, 20, 42, 43] Because in many cases serious mitral regurgitation carries an unfavorable prognosis in patients with KD, surgical intervention should be conducted at the appropriate time.

Long-term results of mitral valve replacement in children have not been favorable[43] because with growth of the child, the valve becomes relatively stenotic and creates a need for long-term anticoagulation. Calcification and rupture of xenograft valves also occur earlier in children. Repair of the valve is therefore desirable whenever feasible. Many patients have associated coronary artery lesions, and simultaneous coronary artery bypass surgery should therefore be performed.

AORTIC REGURGITATION

Persistent aortic regurgitation is an infrequent complication in patients with KD. Coronary artery bypass surgery combined with replacement of the aortic valve has been sporadically reported.[44, 45]

The leaflets of the aortic valve showed fibrous thickening and contraction, which were considered to be the causes of the regurgitation.

LEFT VENTRICULAR ANEURYSM AND CARDIOMYOPATHY SECONDARY TO KAWASAKI DISEASE

A left ventricular aneurysm and diffuse myocardial dysfunction resembling dilated or ischemic cardiomyopathy have been observed as a result of myocardial infarction secondary to coronary artery obstruction or as a result of associated myocarditis in patients with KD. The incidence of myocardial infarction in children as a sequela of KD is relatively high, but the formation of left ventricular aneurysms is extremely rare, presumably because the formation of a coronary artery collateral circulation is much better in children than in adults and a broad transmural infarction producing a left ventricular aneurysm is rare. Surgery should be limited to those with poor collateral vessel formation and significant left ventricular dysfunction caused by an aneurysm or the apparent onset of severe ventricular arrhythmias. Surgical resection of left ventricular aneurysms (aneurysmectomy) and cardiac transplantation for diffuse cardiomyopathy have been successfully performed and reported.[46, 47]

AORTIC AND PERIPHERAL ANEURYSMS

In addition to coronary artery aneurysms, other aneurysms are occasionally observed in the abdominal aorta and the iliac and axillary arteries, nearly always in association with coronary artery aneurysms.[13, 20] Abdominal aneurysms have been repaired by replacement with a graft.[48]

Rupture of such aneurysms (in coronary arteries, the abdominal aorta, or peripheral arteries) has not been reported over the period of convalescence (3 weeks after the acute onset of KD), probably because of the formation of a thickened fibrotic wall of the aneurysm as a result of healing of the inflammation. This is markedly different from generation of the wall of atherosclerotic aneurysms. This fact must be stressed when surgical resection of aneurysms is considered in patients with KD.

REFERENCES

1. Kawasaki T: Acute febrile mucocutaneous syndrome with lymphoid involvement with specific desquamation of the fingers and toes in children (in Japanese). *Jpn J Allergy* 16:178–222, 1967.

2. Kawasaki T, Kosaki I, Okawa S, et al: A new infantile acute febrile mucocutaneous lymph node syndrome (MLNS) prevailing in Japan. *Pediatrics* 54:271–276, 1974.
3. Gersony WM: Kawasaki disease, clinical overview. *Cardiol Young* 1:192–195, 1991.
4. Kitamura S, Kawachi K, Harima R, et al: Surgery for coronary heart disease due to mucocutaneous lymph node syndrome (Kawasaki disease). *Am J Cardiol* 51:444–448, 1983.
5. Kitamura S, Kawashima Y, Kawachi K, et al: Severe mitral regurgitation due to coronary arteritis of mucocutaneous lymph node syndrome, a new surgical entity. *J Thorac Cardiovasc Surg* 80:629–636, 1980.
6. Kato H, Kitamura S, Kawasaki T: Guidelines for treatment and management of cardiovascular sequelae in Kawasaki disease. *Heart Vessels* 3:50–54, 1987.
7. Kitamura S, Kawashima Y, Kawachi K, et al: Left ventricular function in patients with coronary arteritis due to acute febrile mucocutaneous lymph node syndrome or related disease. *Am J Cardiol* 40:156–164, 1977.
8. Chow LT, Chow W, Tse CC, et al: Kawasaki disease—sudden death as the first presenting symptom. *Cardiol Young* 2:73–77, 1992.
9. Furusho K, Kamiya T, Nakano H, et al: High-dose intravenous gammaglobulin for Kawasaki disease. *Lancet* 2:1055–1058, 1984.
10. Newburger JW, Takahashi M, Burns JC: The treatment of Kawasaki syndrome with intravenous gamma-globulin. *N Engl J Med* 315:341–347, 1986.
11. Kitamura S: Surgery for coronary artery disease and pediatric ischemic heart disease due to Kawasaki disease. *Asian Med J* 36:333–340, 1993.
12. Suzuki A, Kamiya T: Visualization of coronary arterial lesions in Kawasaki disease by coronary angiography. *Cardiol Young* 1:225–233, 1991.
13. Naoe S, Shibuya K, Takahashi K, et al: Pathological observations concerning the cardiovascular lesions in Kawasaki disease. *Cardiol Young* 1:212–220, 1991.
14. Kato H, Ichinose E, Yoshioka F, et al: Fate of coronary aneurysms in Kawasaki disease: Serial coronary angiography and long term follow up study. *Am J Cardiol* 49:1758–1766, 1982.
15. Takahashi M, Mason W, Lewis AB: Regression of coronary aneurysms in patients with Kawasaki syndrome. *Circulation* 75:387–394, 1987.
16. Suma K, Takeuchi Y, Shiroma K, et al: Early and late post-operative studies in coronary arterial lesions resulting from Kawasaki's disease in children. *J Thorac Cardiovasc Surg* 84:224–229, 1982.
17. Kato H, Ichinose E, Kawasaki T: Myocardial infarction in Kawasaki disease, clinical analysis in 195 cases. *J Pediatr* 108:923–927, 1986.
18. Ino T, Akimoto K, Ohkubo M, et al: Application of percutaneous transluminal coronary angioplasty to coronary arterial stenosis in Kawasaki disease. *Circulation* 93:1709–1715, 1996.

19. Tatara K, Murata M, Itoh K, et al: Management of severe coronary sequelae of Kawasaki disease. *Am Heart J* 131:576–581, 1996.

20. Kitamura S: Surgical management for cardiovascular lesions in Kawasaki disease. *Cardiol Young* 1:240–253, 1991.

21. Kitamura S, Kawashima Y, Fujita T, et al: Aortocoronary bypass grafting in a child with coronary artery obstruction due to mucocutaneous lymph node syndrome: Report of a case. *Circulation* 53:1035–1040, 1976.

22. Kitamura S, Kameda Y, Seki T, et al: Long-term outcome of myocardial revascularization in patients with Kawasaki coronary artery disease. *J Thorac Cardiovasc Surg* 107:663–674, 1994.

23. Kitamura S, Kawachi K, Oyama C, et al: Severe Kawasaki heart disease treated with an internal mammary artery graft in pediatric patients. A first successful report. *J Thorac Cardiovasc Surg* 89:860–866, 1985.

24. Kitamura S, Seki T, Kawachi K, et al: Excellent patency and growth potential of internal mammary artery grafts in pediatric coronary bypass surgery: New evidence for a "live" conduit. *Circulation* 78:129S–139S, 1989.

25. Sandiford FM, Vargo TA, Shin JY, et al: Successful triple coronary artery bypass in a child with multiple coronary aneurysms due to Kawasaki's disease. *J Thorac Cardiovasc Surg* 79:283–287, 1980.

26. Mains C, Wiggins J, Groves B, et al: Successful therapy for a complication of Kawasaki's disease. *Ann Thorac Surg* 35:197–200, 1983.

27. Myers JL, Gleason MM, Cyran SE, et al: Surgical management of coronary insufficiency in a child with Kawasaki's disease: Use of bilateral internal mammary arteries. *Ann Thorac Surg* 46:459–461, 1988.

28. D'Amico TA, Sabiston DC Jr: Kawasaki's disease, in Sabiston DC Jr, Spencer FC (eds): *Surgery of the Chest.* Philadelphia, WB Saunders, 1990, pp 1759–1766.

29. Mavroudis C, Backer CL, Muster AJ, et al: Expanding indications for pediatric coronary artery bypass. *J Thorac Cardiovasc Surg* 111:181–189, 1996.

30. Burns JC, Shike H, Gordon JB, et al: Sequelae of Kawasaki disease in adolescents and young adults. *J Am Coll Cardiol* 28:253–257, 1996.

31. Fujiwara T, Fujiwara H, Nakano H: Pathological feature of coronary arteries in children with Kawasaki disease in which coronary arterial aneurysm was absent at autopsy: Quantative analysis. *Circulation* 78:345–350, 1988.

32. Suzuki A, Kamiya T, Ono Y, et al: Aortocoronary bypass surgery for coronary arterial lesions resulting from Kawasaki disease. *J Pediatr* 116:567–573, 1990.

33. Kitamura S, Kawachi K, Seki T, et al: Bilateral internal mammary artery grafts for coronary bypass operations in children. *J Thorac Cardiovasc Surg* 99:708–715, 1990.

34. Kitamura S, Kawachi K, Seki T, et al: Use of internal thoracic artery

graft in congenital or acquired pediatric coronary artery disease, in Fournial G, Glock Y, Roux D, et al (eds): *Internal Thoracic Artery for Myocardial Revascularization.* Toulouse, France, Imprimeries fournié, 1990, pp 297–304.

35. Takeuchi Y, Gomi A, Okamura Y, et al: Coronary revascularization in a child with Kawasaki disease: Use of right gastroepiploic artery. *Ann Thorac Surg* 50:294–296, 1990.

36. Isomura T, Hisatomi K, Hirano A, et al: The internal thoracic artery and its branches after coronary artery anastomoses in pediatric patients. *J Card Surg* 7:225–230, 1992.

37. Kawachi K, Kitamura S, Seki T, et al: Hemodynamics and coronary blood flow during exercise after coronary artery bypass grafting with internal mammary arteries in children with Kawasaki disease. *Circulation* 84:618–624, 1991.

38. Newburger JW, Sanders SP, Burns JC, et al: Left ventricular contractility and function in Kawasaki syndrome: Effect of intravenous γ-globulin. *Circulation* 79:1237–1246, 1989.

39. Takahashi M: Myocarditis in Kawasaki syndrome: A minor villain? *Circulation* 79:1398–1400, 1989.

40. Cohen AJ, Grishkin BA, Helsel RA, et al: Surgical therapy in the management of coronary anomalies: Emphasis on utility of internal mammary artery grafts. *Ann Thorac Surg* 47:630–637, 1989.

41. Kitamura S, Kawachi K, Nishii T, et al: Internal thoracic artery grafting for congenital coronary malformation. *Ann Thorac Surg* 53:513–516, 1992.

42. Mishima A, Asano M, Saito T, et al: Mitral regurgitation caused by ruptured chordae tendineae in Kawasaki disease. *J Thorac Cardiovasc Surg* 111:895–896, 1996.

43. Takahashi T, Kadoba K, Taniguchi K, et al: Long-term results of surgical treatment for mitral regurgitation with severe left ventricular dysfunction after myocardial infarction caused by Kawasaki disease. *J Thorac Cardiovasc Surg* 111:893–894, 1996.

44. Kasugai T, Onishi K, Kobayashi J, et al: Aortic regurgitation and coronary artery obstruction due to Kawasaki disease, a case report of successful surgical treatment (in Japanese). *J Jpn Assoc Thorac Surg* 35:124–129, 1987.

45. Fukunaga S, Egashira A, Arinaga K, et al: Aortic valve replacement for aortic regurgitation due to Kawasaki disease: Report of two cases. *J Heart Valve Dis* 5:231–234, 1996.

46. Shimakura T, Nakae S, Kawazoe K, et al: Left ventricular aneurysm due to Kawasaki disease: A surgical case report (in Japanese). *Jpn J Pediatr* 19:551–555, 1978.

47. Travaline JM, Hamilton SM, Ringel RE, et al: Cardiac transplantation for giant coronary artery aneurysms complicating Kawasaki disease. *Am J Cardiol* 68:560–561, 1991.

48. Ohashi H, Yamaguchi M, Tachibana H, et al: Abdominal aortic aneurysm due to Kawasaki disease (in Japanese). *Jpn Circ J* 47:108S, 1983.

CHAPTER 11

Arterial Grafts for Coronary Artery Bypass

Noel L. Mills, M.D.
Professor of Surgery, Tulane University School of Medicine, New Orleans, Louisiana

C onduits for coronary artery bypass grafting (CABG) have continued to be in a state of evolution since the first coronary artery bypass was performed in a human in New York on May, 2, 1961.[1] The saphenous vein graft became the standard conduit by which all graft performance was measured. In the early years, many of the basic technical challenges of CABG were addressed and solved by using the greater saphenous vein. Within 10 years, however, it became apparent that vein grafts in the majority of patients have a very limited longevity.[2, 3] The result was a surge of interest in the internal thoracic artery (ITA). This conduit rapidly became the "gold standard" by which today and probably through the year 2000 all other conduits will be compared. Artificial grafts have failed miserably. Endothelial seeding of artificial grafts, even though successful in experimental animals, has not met with acceptable success for clinical use in humans. A new Gore-Tex graft that offers improved patency by its nature as an arteriovenous fistula warrants close scrutiny. Although there is currently interest in an "all arterial conduit coronary bypass operation,"[4, 5] practicing cardiac surgeons should certainly not apologize for using an ITA to the left anterior descending (LAD) artery combined with saphenous vein grafts to the remaining stenotic coronary arteries as their standard coronary artery bypass operation. Clearly, there is some downside to using any conduit we have available today.

PATENCY

The single biggest problem in assessing any graft in the coronary position is that of obtaining a cineangiographic restudy in such a cost-containing environment. Even academic institutions pursuing important information about this subject find it nearly impossible to perform timely postoperative angiographic studies. Another problem is the way graft patency is reported for patients who have had restudies. "String signs" seen on angiography, even in ITA grafts, are not reported in the literature as "patent grafts." One possible solution would be to distinguish grafts that have "perfect patency" from those reported as having "imperfect patency." Early reports of cardiac valve surgery were complicated by different reporting methods and techniques (often to favorably skew results). This was addressed by the profession so that today there are clear guidelines for reporting valve surgery data. Improvements are needed in the reporting of patency of coronary bypass conduits.

PREPARATION OF GRAFTS

The literature about the preparation of bypass grafts is quite extensive and is beyond the scope of this chapter. However, several important facts have been learned.[6] First, it is clear that the solution for preparation should have a pH close to 7.4. Overdistension of conduits during that preparation is clearly damaging to the intima, so devices have been invented to protect grafts from undue distension. This author is routinely amazed when visiting various operating rooms at the amount of stretching and misuse carried out when grafts are harvested. That part of the operation is often relegated to the least experienced of the operating team. Heat and stretch injuries with or without avulsion of small side branches and/or dissection resulting in poor flow are common ways that ITA grafts are injured. Since the early 1970s, the technique of intraluminal papaverine preparation of arterial grafts has been used by surgeons in New Orleans in more than 10,000 patients with no adverse effects associated with the technique. Body-temperature papaverine solution is left in the graft during pericardiotomy and cannulation. Blood buffers negate any concern regarding the acidic pH of the papaverine solution, which is no lower than that of normal saline. Optical magnification is used to ensure that the 1-mm olive-tipped needle is within the true lumen of the graft. Careful aspiration of blood before injection ensures against injury to the graft. Measurement of free flow from ITA grafts is believed to be mandatory. This test should be routine for all surgeons using ITA grafts because this simple maneuver leaves no question of the adequacy of flow. If a minimum of 120 mL/min is not achieved at a time when systemic blood pressure is 100 mm Hg, there is a problem with the graft. Disease, technical error, and/or conduit injury may result in low free flow. Flow measurement studies of several hundred ITA grafts prepared as described resulted in an average flow of 195 mL/min. "Inadequate flow" of a carefully dissected ITA graft after cardiopulmonary bypass has not been observed when the technique of intraluminal preparation and measurement of free flow has been used. When gentle hydrostatic dilatation is also used, we have found ITA ring segments to be angioparalyzed (unpublished data). A larger, spasm-free distal graft is less prone to technical anastomotic error. It is important to carefully analyze the technique of graft preparation outlined by the authors in any report of coronary grafts because the methods used may be directly responsible for the positive or negative results.

ELECTROCAUTERY

Heat injury to arterial grafts may not be recognized until relatively late postoperatively. Electrocautery injury to radial artery grafts is one of the reasons why that conduit failed as a bypass graft in the early years. Heat injury is one of the most common causes of the "string sign" of ITA grafts. The crest factor of an electrocautery is derived by dividing the voltage peak by the mean squared voltage root and is a measurement of the dissipation of heat energy into the tissues. A low crest factor of less than 8 is unsatisfactory because of heat buildup. The optimal crest factor should be in the range of 10 or 11. Most electrosurgical units today have been adjusted to that crest factor. Some electrosurgical units are actually hazardous for use adjacent to the ITA. Microbubbles from the boiling of blood may be observed in the internal thoracic veins. Such localized heating of the blood in the ITA results in separation of the intima and leads to initiation of dissection of the graft by bubbles. The electrosurgical unit should be used at 50 to 60 W in only the coagulation mode during the initial dissection and be applied parallel and along the sides of the ITA. When actual dissection close to the ITA itself is begun, the coagulation mode of the electrosurgical unit is reduced to 25 to 30 W. Tissue temperatures measured with a myocardial temperature probe adjacent to the ITA during harvest are surprisingly high. Endothelial cell dysfunction occurs to some degree from the dissection itself, and certainly heat injury to this important cell layer must be avoided.

LIPID CONTROL

Venous grafts are particulary susceptible to an adverse lipid environment. Surgeons must monitor patients postoperatively to ensure that they have adequate lipid control. Vein grafts have a significantly increased patency rate when lipids are carefully managed. Hepatic hydroxymethylglutaryl coenzyme A reductase inhibitors not only have salutatory effects because of their antilipid properties but also have a beneficial effect on the blood vessels themselves. To date, there have been few studies concerning antilipid therapy and arterial grafts. The ITA is resistant to lipid invasion, presumably because of its unique endothelial cell function. Postoperative CABG results are more than ever being scrutinized, and they are being compared with the results of percutaneous transluminal coronary angioplasty and stents with regard to quality of life, morbidity and mortality, and cost analysis. It behooves the surgeon to play an active role in ensuring that the postoperative patient has optimal antiplatelet and antilipid treatment to aid in maximizing long-term graft patency.

PROXIMAL ATTACHMENT OF THE ARTERIAL CONDUIT

The pedicle internal thoracic graft avoids a proximal surgical connection and the inherent technical pitfalls that may be incurred. However, there is an incidence of atherosclerosis of approximately 3% at the subclavian-ITA junction. This author and other surgeons have occasionally had to perform a subclavian carotid bypass in patients with a functioning ITA graft to the LAD in whom symptoms developed as the subclavian stenosis became significant in the ensuing years after the coronary bypass. Because of this incidence of proximal ITA disease, it is again emphasized that surgeons ensure that the ITA has adequate free flow (a minimum of 120 mL/min).

Inferior epigastric grafts, radial artery grafts, etc., all require proximal attachment. Techniques for this include anastomosis of the proximal arterial bypass conduit to the hood of a saphenous vein graft, anastomosis to a 1- to 2-cm circular pericardial patch on the aorta, or a direct anastomosis to the aorta itself. In general, arterial free conduits anastomosed to the aorta have a significantly lower patency rate than do pedicle ITA grafts. How much of this is due to technical factors and how much is a result of physiologic alterations are uncertain. However, the dp/dt of the ascending aorta is much greater than that of second-generation arteries, e.g., the ITA. Increased dp/dt has been proposed to result in a hyperplastic process at the proximal aortic anastomotic site. It has therefore been recommended that free arterial grafts be anastomosed to the upper third of the ITA as an inverted "Y" to avoid this problem (Fig 1). Some proponents of the technique theorize that the improved patency is due to the acute angle of the graft origin from

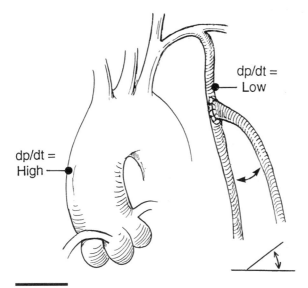

FIGURE 1.

The ascending aorta has a higher dp/dt than do second-generation arteries (e.g., the internal thoracic artery [ITA]). It has been theorized that the higher dp/dt is responsible for the hyperplastic process that can cause failure of free grafts anastomosed to the ascending aorta. Some surgeons are recommending that free arterial conduits be anastomosed to second-generation arteries such as the ITA, as seen in this diagram. The acute angle of origin of the graft from the ITA has also been offered as explanation for the improved patency with this technique. This is one of the more important concepts to recently arise in the field of coronary bypass and is presently being investigated further in a number of centers.

the ITA as opposed to the nearly 90-degree angle of grafts arising from the aorta. With this approach, however, one is then relying on multiple areas of the heart being revascularized with a single source of blood supply. A small number of these patients will be at increased risk because of proximal subclavian or ITA atherosclerosis. Presently, several centers are carrying out studies using various free arterial conduits anastomosed to a pedicle ITA as their primary operative technique.

One particular problem is that of performing a proximal free arterial conduit anastomosis to the aorta during the course of a repeat coronary artery bypass. Often, these aortas have a significant degree of fibrosis and thickening. Clearly there is an increased chance of technical mishap in this setting. Surgeons would be well advised to perform the proximal anastomosis to an ITA or subclavian artery.

THE INTERNAL THORACIC ARTERY

Routine use of the ITA among cardiac surgeons has risen from 3% in the early 1970s to above 99% in the 1990s. It stands alone from all other grafts by the fact that it is very resistant to atherosclerosis. Whether this is due to its blood supply from vasa vasorum, its perivascular lymphatic drainage, its well-developed internal elastic membrane, the rare presence of small amounts of smooth muscle cells in the media, or its biochemical difference remains unknown. In general, the ITA is used with no age restriction; however, its use is temporized by cases that are extremely urgent and patients who have a very limited longevity.[7] A number of unresolved problems are discussed in cardiac surgery circles. Use of the ITA in a setup where there will be competition of flow with a larger, shorter saphenous vein graft or a minor native artery stenosis is debated. An extremely thick left ventricle has been a contraindication to ITA use. In severe diabetics, bilateral devascularization of the sternum from internal mammary artery harvest has resulted in an incidence of sternal wound problems of approximately 8.5%. Therefore, it is advised that skeletonized grafts be used as opposed to pedicle grafts in that setting. Spasm proximal to a large pericardiophrenic artery or lateral costal artery origin resulting in low flow remains a problem. When recognized, this situation has been handled by ligating the appropriate vessels to avoid runoff of the intraluminal dilating agent in that section of the ITA. Another technique to differentiate spasm from atherosclerosis is to very carefully introduce a Parsonnet probe (that has been heated in body-temperature saline with the stylet removed) retrogradely across the proximal ITA/subclavian junction. If there is excellent free flow after preparation and harvest and yet the patient has an ipsilateral subclavian bruit, does one use this ITA as a pedicle or convert it to a free graft? Finally, there is the problem of ITA string signs. The causes of string sign are heat and/or stretch injury, dissection along the graft, competition of flow, severe left ventricular hypertrophy, and anastomotic technical mishaps. A question remains as to whether distal ITA string signs are due to one of the aforementioned problems or to histologic differences in the distal ITA as opposed to the more proximal vessel.

Preparation of this graft is critically important. Topical vasodilators appear to have only a temporary effect. Regardless of whether papaverine, nitroglycerin, calcium antagonists, or enoximone is used, it is clear that the best flows will be achieved by a careful technical protocol using an intraluminal vasodilating agent. Extensive coronary endarterectomy to the LAD artery may be used in conjunction with an ITA graft. A 1-cm arteriotomy is used on the coronary artery, and the ITA is sewn directly to the endarterectomized vessel without a vein hood. Besides having the inherent disadvantages of a saphenous vein, a vein hood increases the internal diameter of the endarterectomized coronary artery to a degree that flow is slowed in that area. If a pedicle ITA is used with an extensive endarterectomy, the free flow should be well above 150 and preferably closer to 200 mL/min. The combination of a vein hood and an ITA with only 120-mL/min free flow to an endarterectomized coronary artery has been unsatisfactory for this author.

Harvest of the ITA without damage to the rib cage is as much an art as a science. Use of a retractor such as the modified Favalaro that can sequentially lift each end of the sternum as the anesthesiologist administers an appropriate relaxing agent has worked extremely well. The anterior diaphragm may be divided from the lower end of the sternum by using electrocautery to release it from the attached costal margin. Two parallel incisions are used along the ITA, and the transverse thoracic muscle is opened inferiorly to identify the distal portion of the ITA. The dissection is begun inferiorly and carried superiorly to sense the "nature of the tissues." If damage is incurred in the inferior portion of the ITA, the graft may still be used as a free graft or sometimes even as a pedicle graft. As the ITA is harvested, the branches are clipped on the pedicle side and divided with the Bovie immediately adjacent to the sternum so that the electrocautery will spark out on the sternal side without heat or electrical damage to the graft itself. In the superior portion of the dissection, the deep layer of the deep cervical fascia is opened. The accompanying internal thoracic vein is easily identified with the artery lying just lateral to it. This approach from a medial to lateral direction results in much less chance of damage to the phrenic nerve.

In experimental animals, ligation of the pericardiophrenic artery has been associated with phrenic nerve paralysis. Comparable human studies have not been performed. In the early years, 6-0 polypropylene suture was used for ITA–coronary artery anastomoses. More recently, all anastomoses have been made with 8-0 polypropylene because smaller suture can achieve a leak-free anastomosis. Suturing of leaks, especially in ITA/LAD anastomoses that are in myocardial tunnels where the LAD is thinner walled, present a hazard to the technical quality of the anastomosis. Black silk suture is left along the medial length of the ITA pedicle to facilitate its immediate identity and preservation should the patient require a reoperation. It is wise to avoid placing a right ITA across the anterior mediastinum. Even with the use of artificial pericardium there is the obvious hazard of repeat sternotomy, which may have to be rapidly performed under emergency conditions. This surgeon has not found that an ITA is inherently "too short" for anastomosis to the LAD artery, even if the anastomosis is performed in the distal third of the LAD. It is extremely rare for an ITA to be "too small," perhaps 1 in 1,000. The excellent clinical outcome and long-term patency of this graft provides a standard to which all other grafts can be compared and should be the mainstay of any cardiac surgeon's coronary artery bypass operation.

THE RADIAL ARTERY

The radial artery has been rejuvenated as a bypass graft.[8-10] During an earlier era, early failure of this conduit resulted from traumatic dissection, mechanical dilatation, and ischemic medial necrosis. Avoiding these factors and using pharmacologic vasodilation have resulted in recent success. One active center is currently evaluating the importance of intraoperative and postoperative diltiazem. Indications for radial artery grafting include patients with diabetes (wherein bilateral ITA grafts may be contraindicated), obesity, poor-quality veins, and especially patients who have had relatively recent surgery with early vein graft failure. Problems associated with radial artery grafting are a need for femoral artery monitoring with the use of bilateral radial arteries, loss of a future dialysis access site, and the possibility of hand ischemia. A small percentage of radial arteries have atherosclerosis.

An inadequate ulnar artery collateral as detected by the Allen test contraindicates removal of the radial artery. Other contraindications are injury during harvest, Raynaud/Burger disease, previous arm arterial catheterization, known subclavian artery stenosis, or the presence of subclavian bruits and certain occupations. Age is not a consideration. The mean length obtainable is 22 cm. The learning curve for reliable use of this graft is considerably less than with some other arterial conduits. The role of the vascular laboratory in studying these conduits is being evaluated in the present cost-conscious medical care environment.

Circumferential arm preparation and a single incision are required. No electrocautery is used once the brachioradialis muscle is exposed and retracted. An en bloc dissection incorporating artery and veins is used. An operative Allen test is performed to confirm adequate collateral circulation after the branches are ligated.

The multibranch area near the elbow and at the wrist are avoided. After distal division just above a significant branch, intraluminal papaverine and/or diltiazem is used, and initial dilatation is achieved with the patients' arterial pressure and the intraluminal drug. The artery is ligated proximally just distal to a significant branch. The antebrachial fascia is not closed, and a noncircumferential dressing is used. The extremity is evaluated just before leaving the operating room. Phlebotomy and pressure cuffs on the arm are avoided postoperatively.

Early radial artery graft patency appears to be comparable to that of the saphenous vein graft. Whether this particular graft will be resistant to graft atherosclerosis on long-term follow-up studies remains to be determined. Questions concerning the subsequent development of ipsilateral subclavian stenosis and ipsilateral ulnar arterial atherosclerosis after radial artery harvest remain to be answered. The effects of IV solutions in the patient's ipsilateral arm circulation are undetermined.

RIGHT GASTROEPIPLOIC ARTERY

The right gastroepiploic artery (RGEA) was used only once in the early years of coronary artery bypass. There was a large hiatus until the late 1980s, when a number of investigators began using that graft. This was prompted by recognition of the limited longevity of venous conduits for coronary bypass grafting. Experience with this graft has been quite extensive in a number of centers, yet other centers have avoided it. This probably relates in part to the increased time required for harvest and the heart surgeon's reluctance to enter the abdomen. Many surgeons have turned to use of the radial artery, which although an adequate conduit, may have higher liability when certain complications occur (e.g., hand ischemia and loss of tissue). The RGEA arises from the gastroduodenal branch of the hepatic artery, a major branch of the celiac axis. The incidence of atherosclerosis in abdominal aortic branches in patients who are candidates for RGEA bypass is unknown, but it is probably relatively uncommon. Patients who undergo an RGEA coronary bypass graft should at least have a stethoscope placed on the abdomen to detect abdominal bruits. At present, there is no reliable way to rule out significant celiac axis atherosclerosis such as exists for ITA grafts (comparison of arm blood pressure measurements). If a significant abdominal bruit is found in the region of the celiac axis, the patient should have an angiogram to ensure that there is no stenosis in the system supplying the RGEA, or the RGEA should be used as a free graft.

Complications with use of the RGEA have been minimal, and generally patients are able to take food and fluids the day after surgery. Pancreatitis is also rare, especially if the dissection is terminated in the RGEA proximal to the origin of the gastroduodenal artery. Abdominal surgery after the RGEA has been used as a bypass graft has not been a major problem. General surgeons should be alerted by the patients or their families that an RGEA has been used. The practice of making a sketch of the bypass graft configuration and providing that to the patient or family in the postoperative period with the admonition to show this to all future doctors can avoid a host of problems and has met with wide acceptance from physicians and families. This author has knowledge of one surgeon who divided a 2.5-mm–diameter RGEA during abdominal surgery. The artery was easily repaired by an end-to-end anastomosis.

The major pitfall in performing an RGEA-to–coronary artery bypass is incurring a twist of the graft. Landmarks are few, and in most patients the graft pedicle is quite fatty. The RGEA is a vessel that has a great tendency to spasm.[11, 12] In a number of aspects, knowledge about this graft is lacking. When the gastroepiploic artery (GEA) is used as a free graft, there may be an even greater tendency to spasm. Some studies show that the GEA changes its size with the patient's alimentation. There is question, therefore, as to whether these grafts should be denervated at the proximal pedicle. Most centers have found that this graft is best suited for bypass to branches to the right coronary artery system. Because atherosclerosis has a propensity to form in the right coronary artery–posterior descending junction, it is preferable to anastomose the graft to the posterior descending artery itself and not the main right coronary artery. Because of the thinness of the RGEA in its distal segment, it is important to use an RGEA graft where it has at least a 2-mm–diameter lumen at the anastomotic site. This is true even if the recipient vessel is smaller in caliber. When 1.5-mm GEA vessels are sutured to coronary arteries, there is a tendency to kink and stenose at the anastomotic neck because of the size of the pedicle that carries the thin-walled vessel. Late studies show that RGEA grafts performed at centers with considerable experience have at least the same early and midterm patency rates as vein grafts. There does not seem to be a propensity for this graft to become atherosclerotic, although late studies are lacking.

INFERIOR EPIGASTRIC ARTERY

The inferior epigastric artery (IEA) was first used as an alternative bypass conduit in 1988. One advantage of this arterial graft, which arises from the inferior end of each external iliac artery just above the inguinal ligament, is that it is bilateral and thus provides two segments of conduit. However, length is limited to approximately 11–13 cm. The artery is more muscular than the ITA and has less elastic lamella in the media. Atherosclerosis is usually not appreciated on angiography, but occasionally at surgery atherosclerosis is seen in the first 1–3 cm of the IEA. Abdominal wall ischemia and hematoma are unusual, yet are specific complications associated with harvest of this graft. Surgical drainage of the paramedian hockey stick incision area is mandatory.

From the paramedian incision, two approaches to the IEA have been used: one is lateral to the artery with the rectus muscle retracted medially, and the other is a medial approach whereupon the rectus muscle is retracted laterally. The medial approach better preserves the nerve supply to the rectus area. In approximately 3% of attempted IEA harvests, the artery is found to be small, fibrotic, and thereby unsatisfactory. The internal diameter of the graft ranges from 2.5 to 3.5 mm proximally and 1.5 to 2.5 mm distally. By nature of its location, this graft has to be used as a free graft. The patency rate has reportedly been improved by anastomosing the proximal graft to a vein patch on the ascending aorta.

The patency rate has ranged from 60% to 85% from 1 to 6 months. Patency has improved when this graft is used as an inverted "Y" graft with proximal anastomosis to an ITA. This author at the present time considers the inferior epigastric artery to be a reasonable alternative graft when another conduit is not feasible or available. It certainly should be considered only after ITAs, the RGEA, and radial arteries have been exhausted. Long-term evaluation to prove its efficacy is not yet available. Its use should be confined to coronary arteries of lesser importance, not, for example, the LAD artery.

RARELY USED ARTERIAL GRAFTS

A number of additional arteries in humans that are expendable may be used in specific rare circumstances. The susceptibility to atherosclerotic changes in these grafts is unknown, and long-term follow-up of a sufficient number of patients is totally lacking. Nonetheless, awareness of these grafts and how to use them can be extremely beneficial to surgeons when there is a challenge in obtaining an adequate amount of conduit for revascularization.

SPLENIC ARTERY

In the early 1970s, the splenic artery was occasionally used for coronary revascularization. It rapidly fell into disfavor because of the tedious technique of dissecting it from the pancreas. Many small branches to the body of the pancreas had to be ligated. A discouraging frequency of atherosclerosis has been found in the splenic artery at autopsy, and the artery is a very tortuous vessel with many fibrous bands. Pancreatitis sometimes occurs after its use, and the friability of the artery plus the calcifications sometimes encountered has led to an abandonment of its use except in unusual circumstances.[13] No angiographic follow-up has been longer than 2 years. On occasion, the splenic artery has provided graft material for patients who have had multiple coronary artery bypass operations when all other graft sources were previously used.

SUBSCAPULAR ARTERY

The subscapular artery arises from the axillary artery, gives off a circumflex scapular branch, and descends along the border of the latissimus dorsi as the dorsal thoracic artery. Postmortem cadaver studies have revealed that 8% of subscapular arteries have significant atherosclerosis. This graft is useful when a patient is having a reoperative coronary bypass via a left lateral thoracotomy. When used as a free graft, the subscapular artery is anastomosed to the descending aorta. On one of six occasions that this author attempted the use of this graft, it was found to be less than 2.0 mm in internal diameter. Excellent patency has been demonstrated by postoperative angiography in the longest follow-up, which is over 4 years. As with other patients who have free arterial grafts, a calcium channel blocker is administered postoperatively. The artery can be exposed to its origin without superior extension of the midline thoracotomy incision, which was used in the first two cases.

LATERAL COSTAL ARTERY

A lateral costal artery is present as a branch of the ITA in approximately 25% of cadavers studied. If this artery reaches the sixth intercostal space, it has sufficient length to be used as a pedicle graft. It is very similar histologically to the ITA; rare fenestrations of the internal elastic membrane are thought to protect against atherosclerosis. It is harvested as a pedicle graft with its venae comitantes as it courses along the midaxillary line. Exposure is facilitated by reducing the tidal volume after opening the left pleura through the median sternotomy incision. The rarity of this artery's use probably relates to the fact that the ITA is not usually studied by preoperative angiography, as well as failure to appreciate its presence. It is useful when there is a paucity of graft material because it can be used to bypass the proximal diagonal, ramus marginalis (intermedius), and high first circumflex marginal coronary branches. It may also be used as an inverted artificial "Y" graft from the ITA pedicle. To date no late-patency studies have been performed.[14] From its embryology and histologic appearance, however, this artery would be expected to behave as an ITA.

THE LEFT GASTRIC ARTERY

Three patients in Cincinnati have undergone CABG with the left gastric artery. This branch of the hepatic artery was dissected out from along the lessor curvature of the stomach and brought through a diaphragmatic window as a pedicle graft in two patients. It was used as an inverted "Y" graft from the ITA in a third patient. Two patients with early angiographic studies showed perfect patency. The third patient succumbed to lung cancer 1 year postoperatively and was found to have a patent graft. The left gastric artery usually has many branches, which may limit the length of this conduit. Reports of the physiology and histology of this conduit are not available.

LATERAL FEMORAL CIRCUMFLEX

Use of the descending branch of the lateral femoral circumflex artery has recently been reported from Japan.[15] Angiography revealed perfect patency 10 days postoperatively. The deep muscular location of this artery makes it less appealing as a bypass graft. This early experience should be kept in mind if one is really struggling to obtain enough conduit; however, there have been no histologic or physiologic studies concerning the use of this artery as a coronary bypass graft.

SYNTHETIC GRAFTS

Artificial grafts are rarely used for coronary bypass. Knitted or woven Dacron grafts are associated with early occlusion, and the patency rate of polytetrafluoroethylene (PTFE) grafts, even in best of circumstances (short graft and large coronary), is in the range of 15% at 1 year.[16] In some individuals who have diseased vein or lack of native conduit, a synthetic graft may be the only feasible alternative. Indeed, the rare patient may have absolute contraindications to saphenous vein harvest. Development of the Perma-Flow graft (Possis Medical, Inc., Minneapolis) was based on a concept from Italy; using the saphenous vein as an anteriovenous fistula from the ascending aorta in 12 patients.[17] The graft is allowed to course around the heart with sequential anastomoses being made to stenotic coronary arteries. Finally, the vein graft is anastomosed to the superior vena cava and narrowed with a suture to prevent an arteriovenous fistula overload. The Perma-Flow graft is a PTFE conduit that is also implanted as an arteriovenous graft. In the distal portion of the graft, there is a Venturi restrictor that controls the flow to less than 10% of the cardiac output, thereby preventing high-output cardiac failure. The throat of the graft in the restrictor at the distal end is approximately 1.7 mm in diameter. The reducer cone has a 37-degree angle, and the diffuser cone in the distal part of the restrictor segment has an angle of 14 degrees, both of which are dynamically important to limit flow and maintain arterial backpressure (Fig 2). Over 50 Perma-Flow grafts have been implanted in the United States since 1992, many in desperate situations. Thirty-day and 1-year catheterizations were required in the Food and Drug Administration (FDA)–approved protocol; however, data have remained elusive because many patients who are doing well refuse repeat angiography. Anticoagulation has not been used uniformly, and all patients have been taking aspirin daily. Bypass to the LAD artery has been avoided in most of these patients. Postoperative catheterization from 1 week to 9 months in 28 patients with 67 anastomoses at risk revealed a 97% patency rate. Ten patients with 20 eligible anastomoses studied at 4–38 months had 18 patent anastomoses (90%). The postoperative patency rate of this graft appears to approach that of vein grafts. This graft material is technically difficult to work with, especially because the FDA has approved only the thicker PTFE graft material (0.42 mm). Careful graft alignment is mandatory to prevent kinking during cardiac contractions. A transverse orientation of the graft across two adjacent recipient coronary arteries with both anastomoses at right angles may result in tension and kinking during the cardiac cycle because of the inelasticity of the graft material.

A second synthetic graft (THORATEC, Berkeley, Calif) is made from polyurethane BPS-215M. It is an elastomeric biomaterial that contains a unique surface-modifying additive for improved biocompatibility. These 2- to 3.5-mm grafts have three layers, each with different properties to make the graft resemble natural arteries. They have been implanted in 27 patients in Canada and Germany. Five deaths have occurred from causes unrelated to the grafts. Twenty-two of the patients are asymptomatic as of December 1996, and the longest patient follow-up is over 3 years. The graft is used as a standard saphenous graft from the aorta directly end to side to the coronary artery.

These works must be carefully monitored, for with improved pharmacologic management of platelet activity and the clotting process, the success rate may be improved to the point that

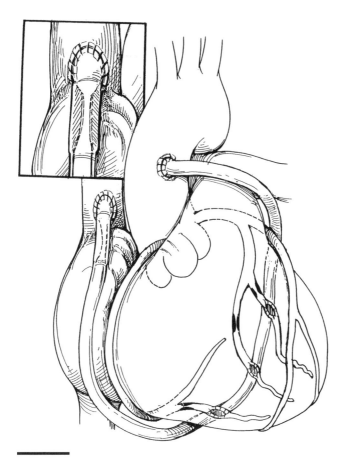

FIGURE 2.

The Perma-Flow polytetrafluoroethylene (PTFE) prosthetic coronary by-pass graft has demonstrated an acceptable early success rate. An arterio-venous (AV) fistula is formed by the conduit between the ascending aorta and the superior vena cava. There is a Venturi flow restrictor at the ve-nous end of the conduit. The throat segment of the Venturi flow restrictor is 1.7 mm in diameter, which allows a flow of approximately 500 mL/min. This prevents an overload from the AV fistula. Backpressure is generated proximal to the restrictor area of the graft to encourage blood pressure fa-vorable for coronary flow. The superior vena cava anastomosis is per-formed first. The length of PTFE between the Venturi flow restrictor area of the graft and the superior vena cava is kept very short. As the graft is laid around the heart, the number of sequential anastomoses necessary are made between the graft and the appropriate coronary artery. Finally, the proximal part of the graft is anastomosed to the ascending aorta.

such grafts will be indicated more frequently in coronary bypass surgery.

ILLUSTRATIVE CASES

Six cases are presented that represent complex challenges for coronary revascularization (Figs 3–8). The solutions for these individual patients are not offered as the only way to manage the problems. They are techniques that have been used by this author and resulted in all patients surviving without any major complications.

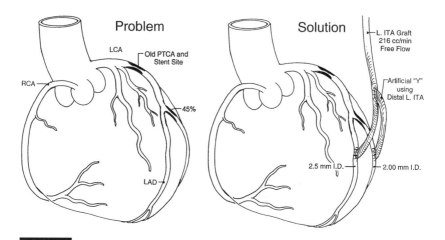

FIGURE 3.

A, problem. A 38-year-old male has hyperhomocystinemia, an elevated low-density lipoprotein (LDL) concentration, and a high-grade proximal left anterior descending *(LAD)* artery stenosis. Greater than a 60-degree angle is found between the LAD and diagonal, which makes a sequential anastomosis undesirable because of the risk of a possible kink. The 45% stenosis present in the proximal large diagonal is prone to competition of flow with a left internal thoracic artery *(L. ITA)* should a vein graft be used to that diagonal.

B, solution. Extra length of the distal segment of the L. ITA is retained for anastomosis to itself proximally to form an artificial "Y" configuration before cardiopulmonary bypass. The "parent graft" is anastomosed to the LAD artery, and the artificial "Y" limb is anastomosed to the diagonal branch. Because the LAD artery bypass is the more important, it would be unwise in this situation to perform a sequential anastomosis because of the wide angle between the LAD and the diagonal, which is a setup for a graft kink upon refilling of the heart and cessation of cardiopulmonary bypass. Postoperatively, this type of patient is treated with folic acid and B vitamins for hyperhomocystinemia in addition to a hepatic hydroxymethylglutaryl coenzyme A reductase inhibitor for his elevated LDL. *Abbreviations: RCA,* right coronary artery; *LCA,* left coronary artery; *PTCA,* percutaneous transluminal coronary angioplasty; *I.D.,* internal diameter.

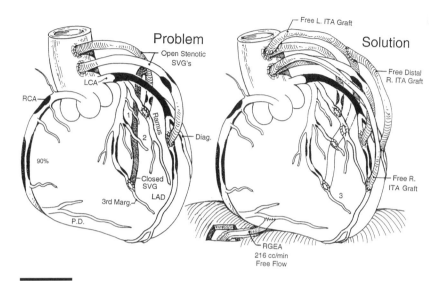

FIGURE 4.

A, problem. A 67-year-old physician has a left main coronary occlusion and two open, but stenotic saphenous vein grafts *(SVGs)* to the left anterior descending *(LAD)* artery and ramus marginalis. There is disease in the LAD artery distal to the vein graft anastomosis and significant circumflex stenosis. The patient has bilateral subclavian artery stenoses and a femoral-femoral bypass graft. He is living off of the stenotic SVGs and a severely stenotic right coronary artery *(RCA)*. The ascending aorta is somewhat thickened and scarred from the previous operation. He previously had severe phlebitis in the remaining leg vein and inadequate revascularization of that leg by the femoral-femoral graft.

  B, solution. Previous phlebitis and poor blood supply contraindicate any attempt at vein harvest from that leg. The left and right internal thoracic arteries *(L. ITA and R. ITA)* are used as free grafts because of the subclavian stenoses. The proximal R. ITA segment is used to bypass the LAD. The distal R. ITA graft is used as an artificial "Y" graft to the diagonal. A pedicle right gastroepiploic artery *(RGEA)* graft bypasses the posterior descending *(P.D.)* artery. The free L. ITA graft revascularizes the ramus marginalis, a medium-sized second marginal, and the large third marginal branch. Radial artery grafts are contraindicated because of the subclavian stenoses. The free grafts are anastomosed to the disease-free hood of the SVGs to avoid suturing a free graft to a thickened aorta. The stenotic SVG to the LAD artery is left untouched.

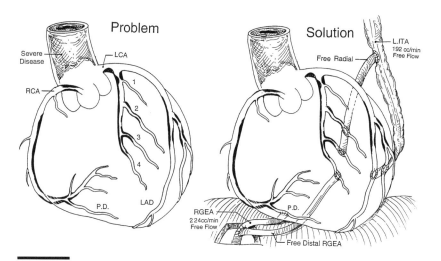

FIGURE 5.

A, problem. A 70-year-old female patient had angina decubitus and eventration of the left diaphragm. She has a porcelain aorta secondary to atherosclerosis and a critical left main stenosis. The patient is obese with ulcerated, edematous legs. Previously, the patient had bilateral complete vein stripping. She has severe diabetes and mild mitral regurgitation.

   B, solution. A "no-touch technique" is used for the operation with hypothermic intermittent low-flow cardiopulmonary bypass and fibrillatory arrest during the anastomoses. The right gastroepiploic artery *(RGEA)* and radial artery are used to avoid bilateral internal thoracic artery (ITA) grafts in this diabetic lady with an osteoporotic sternum. The RGEA was long enough to be used for two bypasses with a direct anastomosis to the posterior descending *(P.D.)* artery and a "Y" graft to the 2-mm (internal diameter) fourth marginal branch. The left ITA *(L.ITA)* was used sequentially to bypass the diagonal and the left anterior descending *(LAD)* artery. A free radial graft is used as an inverted "Y" graft to the second and third marginal. This was anastomosed to the underside of the L.ITA graft. Conduit lengths are measured with umbilical tape marked at 5-cm intervals with a sterile marking pen. The "Y" anastomoses are performed before instituting cardiopulmonary bypass. The "no-touch technique" avoids the problem of embolic debris from the aorta and the undesirability of suturing an arterial graft to a Dacron graft after replacement of a diseased segment of the ascending aorta. The eventration was plicated before cessation of cardiopulmonary bypass. *Abbreviations: RCA,* right coronary artery; *LCA,* left coronary artery.

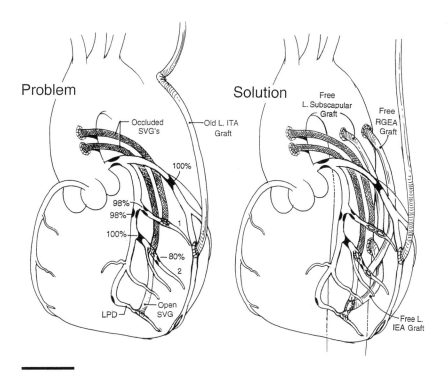

FIGURE 6.

A, problem. A 63-year-old male draftsman has a left main stenosis and is undergoing a fourth coronary artery bypass. There is a functioning left internal thoracic artery *(L. ITA)* with a 70% stenotic kink at the junction of its upper and middle third. There is a dominant left coronary artery, and the patient has no greater or lessor saphenous vein. On angiography, the L. ITA is seen adhered to the posterior of the sternum on the lateral view, and on the anteroposterior view in one area it is found under the midline of the sternum. Previous vein grafts to the first marginal and second marginal–left posterior descending *(LPD)* artery are occluded. Both radial arteries had been used for monitoring purposes many times and arterial pulses at the wrist were reduced.

    B, solution. A left thoracotomy is performed for the operation and a free left subscapular artery graft is harvested and used to revascularize the 2.5-mm first marginal branch. A free right gastroepiploic artery *(RGEA)* is used to bypass the second marginal. The incision used to harvest a left inferior epigastric artery *(L. IEA)* graft is extended inferiorly to expose the left femoral vessels for cannulation. The L. ITA is dissected out proximally to eliminate the kink. The free L. IEA graft is anastomosed to the old, open, nondiseased segment of the previously placed vein graft between the second marginal and the LPD artery. The RGEA and subscapular artery grafts are anastomosed to the descending aorta superior to the hilum of the lung, and the IEA graft is placed inferior to the hilum. *Abbreviation: SVG,* saphenous vein graft.

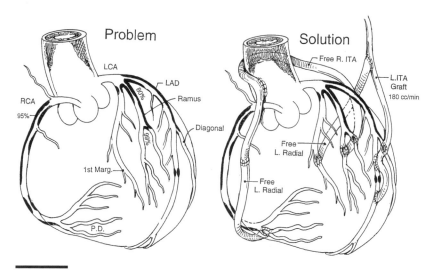

FIGURE 7.

A, problem. A 58-year-old male patient needs six bypasses and is a severe insulin-dependent diabetic. He had previously undergone aortoiliac and bilateral femoral distal bypass and has had loss of his toes. There is a severe stenosis affecting all major coronary arteries, a right lung lesion, and the ascending aorta is partially diseased. He had undergone a gastrectomy for ulcer.

B, solution. A double sequential left internal thoracic artery *(L.ITA)* was used to revascularize the anterior of the left ventricle by bypassing the major diagonal and the lesion at the junction of the middle and lower third of the left anterior descending *(LAD)* artery. Half of the left radial artery conduit was used for the distal circumflex bypass. This was anastomosed proximally to the L.ITA to form an inverted "Y" graft. The right internal thoracic artery *(R. ITA)* was used to bypass two branches of the ramus marginalis and then passed through the transverse sinus to be anastomosed side to side to a disease-free area of the ascending aorta. The second half of the radial artery graft was anastomosed end to end to the free R. ITA graft to provide sufficient length of conduit for bypass to the posterior descending *(P.D.)* coronary artery. Use of the inferior epigastric artery was contraindicated because of significant abdominal aortic, femoral, and distal arterial disease. Removal of vein below the knee was also contraindicated. The prior gastrectomy eliminated the right gastroepiploic artery. The diseased ascending aorta allowed only one anastomosis to be made safely. A 1-cm elliptical aortotomy was used for a long side-to-side anastomosis of the free R. ITA. The free ITA grafts were taken with very conservative use of electrocautery to prevent sternal wound problems. The lung lesion was benign. *Abbreviations: RCA,* right coronary artery; *LCA,* left coronary artery.

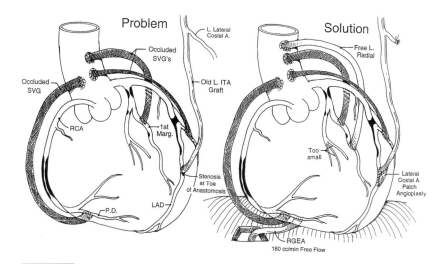

FIGURE 8.

A, problem. A 41-year-old male patient had early saphenous vein graft *(SVG)* occlusions soon after his coronary artery bypass grafting. There is stenosis from technical error at the toe of the left internal thoracic artery *(L. ITA)*–left anterior descending *(LAD)* artery anastomosis. His lipids were well controlled with a "statin" drug and niacin. The homocystine level was 8 (normal, <14). The coagulopathy workup was negative. A left lateral costal artery is seen on postoperative angiography of the L. ITA.

    B, solution. An all-arterial operation is performed to avoid using any SVGs that failed early from unknown causes. A lateral costal artery patch angioplasty is used to reconstruct the stenosed distal L. ITA anastomosis. A free left radial artery graft is used to bypass the first marginal, and a pedicle right gastroepiploic artery *(RGEA)* graft is used to revascularize the posterior descending *(P.D.)* artery. The right internal thoracic artery is preserved for possible use in the future in this young man by using the lateral costal artery, which is histologically similar to the internal thoracic artery. *Abbreviation: RCA,* right coronary artery.

REFERENCES

1. Goetz RH, Rohman M, Haller JD, et al: Internal mammary–coronary artery anastomosis: A nonsuture method employing tantalum rings. *J Thorac Cardiovasc Surg* 41:378–386, 1961.
2. Bryan AJ, Angelini GD: The biology of saphenous vein graft occlusion: Etiology and strategies for prevention. *Curr Opin Cardiol* 9:641–649.
3. Grooters RK, Nishida H: *Alternative Bypass Conduits and Methods for Surgical Coronary Revascularization.* Armonk, NY, Futura Publishing, 1994.
4. Amrani M, El Khoury G, Dion R: Complete myocardial revascularization with arterial grafts without using the mammary artery. *Eur J Cardiothorac Surg* 8:283–284, 1994.

5. Angelini GD, Bryan AI, Dion R: *Arterial Conduits in Myocardial Revascularization.* London, Arnold, 1996.
6. Mills NL, Bringaze WL: Preparation of the internal mammary artery graft: Which is the best method? *J Thorac Cardiovasc Surg* 98:73–79, 1989.
7. Galbut DL, Traad EA, Dorman MJ, et al: Seventeen-year experience with bilateral mammary artery grafts. *Ann Thorac Surg* 49:195–201, 1990.
8. Calafiore AM, DiGimmarco G, Theodori G: Radial artery and inferior epigastric artery as composite graft with an IMA: Improved midterm angiographic results. *Ann Thorac Surg* 60:517–524, 1995.
9. Brodman RF, Frame R, Camacho M, et al: Routine use of unilateral and bilateral radial arteries for coronary artery bypass graft surgery. *J Am Coll Cardiol* 28:959–963, 1996.
10. Acar C, Iebara VA, Portoghese M, et al: Revival of the radial artery for coronary artery bypass grafting. *Ann Thorac Surg* 54:652–660, 1992.
11. Ali AT, Montgomery W, Santamone WP, et al: Protecting the GEA against spasm: Papaverine vs. calcium channel blockers in procine gastroepiploic artery segments. Presented at the 13th Annual Meeting of the Association for Academic Surgery, Chicago, Nov 13–16, 1996.
12. Suma H: Spasm of the gastroepilploic artery graft. *Ann Thorac Surg* 49:168–169, 1990.
13. Mullen DK: Free splenic artery used in aortocoronary bypass. *Ann Thorac Surg* 55:162–163, 1993.
14. Hartman AR, Mawulaude KI, Dervan JP, et al: Myocardial revascularization with the lateral costal artery. *Ann Thorac Surg* 49:816–818, 1990.
15. Takahiko O, Tatsumi MD, Tanaka Y, et al: Descending branch of lateral femoral circumflex artery as a free graft for myocardial revascularization: A case report. *J Thorac Cardiovasc Surg* 111:546–547, 1996.
16. Chard RB, Johnson DC, Nunn GR, et al: Aorto-coronary bypass grafting with polytetrafluoroethylene conduits: Early and late outcomes in eight patients. *J Thorac Cardiovasc Surg* 94:132–134, 1987.
17. Spaminato N, Stassano P: Surgical A-V fistula in aortocoronary snake graft. *J Cardiovasc Surg* 29:100–102, 1988.

CHAPTER 12

Revision of the Traditional Atriopulmonary Fontan Connection

Frank G. Scholl, M.D.
Research Fellow, Division of Cardiothoracic Surgery, UCLA Medical Center, Los Angeles, California

Juan C. Alejos, M.D.
Assistant Professor of Pediatrics, Division of Cardiology, UCLA Medical Center, Los Angeles, California

Hillel Laks, M.D.
Professor and Chief, Division of Cardiothoracic Surgery, UCLA Medical Center, Los Angeles, California

D uring the past 25 years, the modified Fontan procedure has become the procedure of choice for an increasing variety of complex congenital heart defects with a single-ventricle physiology. With the availability of long-term follow-up of patients undergoing the traditional right atrium (RA)-to–pulmonary artery (PA) Fontan connection, it has become evident that there is a significant incidence of certain complications associated with this procedure. These complications include RA dilatation, arrhythmias, atrial thrombosis, and protein-losing enteropathy and are a result of the effects of chronic RA hypertension, turbulent flow, stasis, and elevated systemic venous pressures. Management of these late complications remains challenging because many of them are refractory to medical therapy such as antiarrythmics and anticoagulants or even minimally invasive treatments such as radiofrequency ablation for atrial arrythmias and fibrinolytic therapy for atrial thrombi. Given the failure of medical treatment in many of these cases, a satisfactory solution must come through the use of surgical intervention to alter RA geometry and thus the hemodynamic factors causing these complications.

BACKGROUND

Since its introduction by Fontan and Baudet[1] in 1971, the Fontan operation has undergone a series of technical modifications to minimize the impact of postoperative changes in pulmonary vascular resistance and systemic venous pressure on early survival. The RA-to-PA connection was described by Kreutzer and soon became the standard Fontan connection. It was supplanted by the lateral tunnel or total cavopulmonary connection, which was proposed as a means of reducing turbulence and improving forward flow. There are, however, large numbers of patients who underwent the traditional RA-to-PA connection, and complications related to inclusion of the entire RA in the high-pressure systemic venous system are now developing. Creation of an adjustable intra-atrial communication,[2] baffle fenestration,[3] and exclusion of hepatic venous drainage have all been proposed as solutions to the problems of postoperative low cardiac output and elevated RA pressures.

The long-term complications of the traditional RA-to-PA Fontan connection are significant. Prolonged RA exposure to increased systemic venous pressures leads to RA dilatation. Subsequent hypertrophy of the RA wall results in deep recesses between the trabeculae. This, combined with turbulent flow and areas of stasis, increases the risk of thrombus formation. Right atrial enlargement also results in an increased incidence of atrial arrythmias, including atrial flutter and atrial fibrillation. This also leads to an increased risk of thrombus formation.

The reported incidence of late atrial arrhythmias in patients who have undergone Fontan procedures ranges from 18% to 40%.[4–6] It has been shown that supraventricular arrythmias are more common after the RA-to-PA connection than after the lateral tunnel connection.[6] The pathophysiology of these arrythmias include RA enlargement and RA suture lines that allow for re-entrant arrythmias.[7]

The incidence of atrial arrythmias in patients who also have atrial thrombi or pulmonary emboli has been reported to be 57%.[4] Patients with early atrial thrombi have a notoriously poor outcome. However, those with later atrial thrombi have a more favorable outcome with a greater likelihood of successful treatment.[8]

High systemic venous pressures may eventually lead to hepatic congestion and fibrosis if left unchecked. This may play a role in development of the hypercoaguable state from protein-C deficiency that is seen in some patients after a Fontan operation.[5] Protein-losing enteropathy may also be related to portal venous congestion and to the high systemic venous pressures that result in poor lymphatic drainage from the thoracic duct.[9]

Shielding the RA chamber from high systemic venous pressures and allowing more laminar flow through the atrium may be of benefit in preventing or treating some of these long-term complications. DeLeval and colleagues introduced the concept of the total cavopulmonary connection, which would produce a more laminar pattern of flow and decreased energy dissipation through the dilated contracting RA.[10, 11] In one large series, the cavopulmonary connection or lateral tunnel Fontan connection was associated with a significant reduction in mortality in patients undergoing a "high-risk" Fontan procedure by multivariate analysis.[12]

The lateral tunnel Fontan circulation,[10] by providing more laminar flow, decreasing stasis, and shielding most of the RA from high venous pressures, appears to decrease the incidence of long-term complications. Balaji et al. demonstrated a decreased incidence of early arrythmias and mortality associated with the lateral tunnel Fontan circulation.[13] Gelatt et al. showed a late incidence of atrial tachyarrhythmias of 29% in patients undergoing the traditional Fontan procedure vs. 14% in those undergoing total cavopulmonary connection ($P < 0.02$).[6] In 1993, Paul et al. showed similar results in 45% of their patients who underwent the traditional atriopulmonary connection for late supraventricular arrhythmias and in only 6% of their patients undergoing the total cavopulmonary connection for supraventricular arrhythmias ($P < 0.001$).[14] In a more recent study looking at intermediate-term atrial arrythmias, the lateral tunnel Fontan connection was associated with a lower overall incidence of atrial arrythmias when compared with the atriopulmonary connection at a mean follow-up of 31 months.[15]

Several centers have demonstrated that patients exhibiting some of these long-term complications may benefit from revision of their Fontan circulation. In 1994, Kao[16] reported on three patients who had resolution of their symptoms, which included supraventricular tachycardia and atrial thrombosis, after conversion to a lateral atrial tunnel. More recently, Vitullo et al. reported that patients undergoing revision of Fontan circulation, including conversion to a lateral atrial tunnel or reconnection of their prior Glenn shunt, had a subjective improvement in exercise tolerance and palpitations associated with arrythmias, as well as resolution of protein-losing enteropathy in one patient.[17]

In their report in 1996, Kreutzer and colleagues showed that five of eight patients undergoing lateral tunnel conversion had clinical improvement after short-term follow-up. They believed that conversion was particularly indicated in patients with dilated RAs and pulmonary venous obstruction with symptoms.[18] Revision of the atriopulmonary connection to an intracardiac or extracardiac conduit cavopulmonary connection was used to treat seven patients with pathway obstruction, congestive failure, atrial tachycardias, atrial thrombus, and pulmonary venous obstruction by McElhinney and colleagues. At a median follow-up of 17 months, four of six survivors in the series were functioning at higher New York Heart Association (NYHA) levels than preoperatively, whereas one required cardiac transplantation.[19]

We believe that the advantages of the lateral tunnel are sufficient to warrant revision in patients with refractory atrial arrhythmias, RA dilatation, RA thrombus, or pulmonary venous obstruction secondary to a bulging atrial septum (Fig 1). Additionally, in

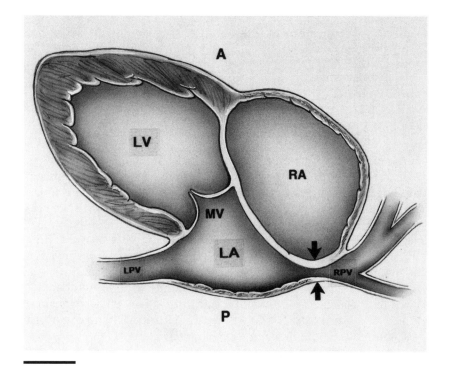

FIGURE 1.

Illustration showing obstruction of the right superior pulmonary vein caused by a bulging intra-atrial septum from a massively dilated right atrium *(RA)*. The view is from the superior aspect of the patient. *Abbreviations: A,* anterior; *LV,* left ventricle; *MV,* mitral valve; *LPV,* left pulmonary vein; *LA,* left atrium; *RPV,* right pulmonary vein; *P,* posterior.

patients with the traditional RA-to-PA connection who require intracardiac repair for other defects such as a restrictive bulboventricular foramen or atrioventricular valve regurgitation, conversion to a lateral tunnel Fontan connection should be considered.

Patients considered for conversion should meet the usual criteria for a Fontan procedure. Those patients with unacceptable pulmonary vascular resistance or poor ventricular function should be considered for heart transplantation.

Surgical options for revision include the creation of an intra-atrial lateral tunnel, intra-atrial inferior vena cava (IVC)–to–superior vena cava (SVC) conduit, or extracardiac conduit. In most cases we have combined these with an adjustable atrial septal defect (ASD) to reduce the systemic venous pressure and optimize cardiac output in the immediate postoperative course.

PROCEDURE

Revision of the traditional RA-to-PA connection is performed as follows. A "redo" median sternotomy is performed, cardiopulmonary bypass is instituted, and blood cardioplegia is achieved. The markedly enlarged RA is opened with a longitudinal incision. Thrombus material, if present, is completely removed. In those patients with an intra-atrial baffle, the previously placed Dacron patch between the systemic venous atrium and the pulmonary venous atrium is completely excised. In other patients, the atrial septum is excised. The atrioventricular valve can be inspected and repaired or replaced if necessary. Also, any other intracardiac defects are repaired at this stage, such as resection of outflow tract stenosis or a restrictive bulboventricular foramen. Usually a bidirectional Glenn shunt is created in the usual fashion, and the distal end of the SVC is sutured to the inferior aspect of the right PA. A 0.8-mm Gore-Tex (W.L. Gore & Associates, Flagstaff, Ariz) patch is used to create a lateral tunnel connecting the orifices of the SVC and IVC. Full-thickness bites are taken to avoid a suture line leak. In some cases we have not divided the SVC to create a Glenn shunt. In this situation the superior end of the tunnel includes both the orifice of the SVC and the previously placed RA-to-PA connection as shown in Figure 2. An adjustable ASD is created along the posterior lateral suture line of the tunnel. The orifice of the coronary sinus remains on the left side of the atrial baffle. After the tunnel is created and the adjustable ASD checked for function, portions of the redundant RA wall are excised. The RA is then closed with a running suture of 4-0 Prolene (Ethicon, Somerville, NJ). Alterna-

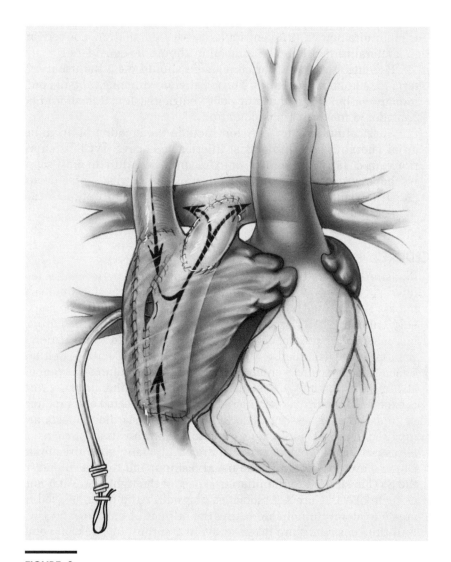

FIGURE 2.

Lateral tunnel Fontan conversion showing modification of the existing right atrium–to–pulmonary artery connection. A 0.8-mm Gore-Tex patch is used to create the lateral tunnel connecting the orifices of the inferior vena cava with both the orifice of the superior vena cava and the previous connection between the right atrium and the pulmonary artery. A snare-controlled, adjustable atrial septal defect is shown along the posterior edge of the lateral tunnel.

tively, a Gore-Tex tube graft can be used to create an intracardiac conduit from the orifice of the IVC to the SVC, as in Figure 3. The redundant RA wall is excised and the atrium is closed. Systemic and pulmonary atrial pressure lines are inserted. Air is removed from the heart, and the patient is weaned from bypass. After coming off bypass, the ASD, which has been left wide open, is slowly constricted by using a snare, with a target arterial oxygen saturation of 85% to 92% on an F_{IO_2} of 100% and a systemic venous pressure of 15 mm Hg or less.

In the patients in whom an extracardiac conduit is used, an adult-sized 18- or 20-mm reinforced Gore-Tex tube graft is interposed between the IVC and the right PA after performing a bidirectional Glenn shunt. An adjustable ASD can be fashioned either by creating a side-to-side window between the functional left atrium and the conduit surrounded by the snare or by inserting a 6- or 8-mm short tube graft between the large tube graft and the lateral atrial wall, as illustrated in Figure 4.

RESULTS

From 1991 to 1996, 12 patients underwent revision of their traditional RA-to-PA Fontan connection at UCLA Medical Center. The mean age of these patients at the time of revision was 13.9 ± 8.5 years, and the mean interval from the initial Fontan procedure to revision was 6.5 ± 3.5 years. Indications for revision were intractable atrial arrhythmias in 9 patients, 3 of whom had significant atrioventricular valve regurgitation, and 3 of whom had RA thrombosis. One patient underwent revision for right-sided pulmonary venous obstruction from massive RA dilation and a bulging atrial septum. Two patients underwent revision at the time of reoperation for a restrictive bulboventricular foramen (1) and severe atrioventricular valve regurgitation (1). Fontan revision was by conversion to a lateral tunnel in 9 patients, with an intra-atrial IVC-to-SVC conduit in 2 and an extracardiac conduit in 1. In 7 patients a snare-controlled, adjustable ASD from the systemic venous connection to the functional left atrium was created. Three patients had construction of a bidirectional Glenn shunt, 3 patients underwent atrioventricular valve repair, and 1 patient had mitral valve replacement. One patient died of respiratory failure 3 months after her revision, for a hospital mortality rate of 8.3% (1/12). There have been no late deaths. Follow-up of 10 of the remaining 11 patients is available. The mean follow-up interval is 26.8 ± 15.6 months, with a mean NYHA class of 1.2 ± 0.4. Of the 9 patients operated

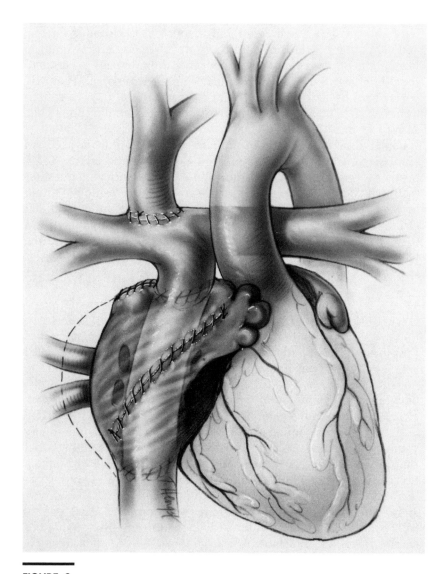

FIGURE 3.

An intracardiac Gore-Tex tube graft total cavopulmonary connection is shown. The tube connects the orifice of the inferior vena cava to the previously placed right atrium–to–pulmonary artery connection. A bidirectional Glenn shunt has been performed. The *dashed line* indicates the redundant portion of the atrial wall, which has been resected before closure of the atriotomy.

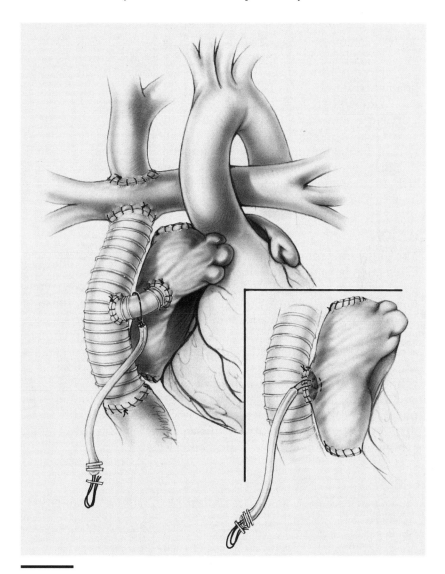

FIGURE 4.

Revision of the Fontan connection by using an extracardiac Gore-Tex ringed conduit with complete takedown of the previously placed traditional right atrium–to–pulmonary artery connection. A bidirectional Glenn shunt has been constructed. Communication has been made between the high-pressure tube graft and the functional left atrium by using an 8-mm Gore-Tex graft. This is controlled by the adjustable snare. The *inset* shows an alternative method in which a direct anastomosis is made between the tube graft and the lateral atrial wall, also controlled with a snare.

on with intractable supraventricular arrhythmias, 7 are well controlled, 1 required radio-frequency atrioventricular node ablation for pacemaker-induced tachycardia, now well controlled, and 1 is having intermittent atrial flutter and is awaiting possible ablation of an aberrant atrial focus.

Postoperatively, anticoagulation in all patients is achieved with warfarin (Coumadin). Patients with an intracardiac tube graft or an extracardiac conduit receive permanent anticoagulation. Those with a lateral tunnel connection undergo anticoagulation for 6 months. If they remain in sinus rhythm and have no further arrhythmias, their treatment is switched to aspirin. There have been no cases of thromboembolism postoperatively.

CONCLUSION

The long-term complications after the traditional RA-to-PA Fontan connection have been well documented. In patients with refractory atrial arrhythmias, RA dilatation, RA thrombus, or pulmonary venous obstruction, conversion to the lateral tunnel modification should be considered. In addition, Fontan patients requiring reoperation for problems such as atrioventricular valve regurgitation or a restrictive bulboventricular foramen should be considered for conversion to a lateral tunnel physiology at the time of their intervention, particularly in the presence of RA dilatation. The early and intermediate results of the conversion to a lateral tunnel–type physiology are favorable, with the majority of patients able to return to an excellent quality of life and the majority of residual symptoms easily controlled with medical therapy.

REFERENCES

1. Fontan F, Baudet E: Surgical repair of tricuspid atresia. *Thorax* 26:240, 1971.
2. Laks H: The partial Fontan procedure: A new concept and its clinical application (editorial). *Circulation* 82:1866–1867, 1990.
3. Bridges ND, Lock JE, Castaneda AR: Baffle fenestration with subsequent transcatheter closure: Modification of the Fontan operation for patients at increased risk (see comments). *Circulation* 82:1681–1689, 1990.
4. Peters NS, Somerville J: Arrhythmias after the Fontan procedure. *Br Heart J* 68:199–204, 1992.
5. Cromme-Dijkhuis AH, Hess J, Hahlen K, et al: Specific sequelae after Fontan operation at mid- and long-term follow-up: Arrhythmia, liver dysfunction, and coagulation disorders. *J Thorac Cardiovasc Surg* 106:1126–1132, 1993.

6. Gelatt M, Hamilton RM, McCrindle BW, et al: Risk factors for atrial tachyarrhythmias after the Fontan operation. *J Am Coll Cardiol* 24:1735–1741, 1994.
7. Gandhi SK, Bromberg BI, Schuessler RB, et al: Characterization and surgical ablation of atrial flutter after the classic Fontan repair. *Ann Thorac Surg* 61:1666–1678, discussion 1678–1679.
8. Fletcher SE, Case CL, Fyfe DA, et al: Clinical spectrum of venous thrombi in the Fontan patient. *Am J Cardiol* 68:1721–1722, 1991.
9. Hess J, Kruizinga K, Bijleveld CM, et al: Protein-losing enteropathy after Fontan operation. *J Thorac Cardiovasc Surg* 88:606–609, 1984.
10. de Leval MR, Kilner P, Gewillig M, et al: Total cavopulmonary connection: A logical alternative to atriopulmonary connection for complex Fontan operations. Experimental studies and early clinical experience (see comments). *J Thorac Cardiovasc Surg* 96:682–695, 1988.
11. DeLeval MR, Bull C, Kilner P: Total cavopulmonary connection: A logical alternative to atriopulmonary connection for complex Fontan operations—experimental studies and early clinical experience. *J Thorac Cardiovasc Surg* 97:636, 1989.
12. Mayer JE Jr, Bridges ND, Lock JE, et al: Factors associated with marked reduction in mortality for Fontan operations in patients with single ventricle. *J Thorac Cardiovasc Surg* 103:444–451, discussion 451–452, 1992.
13. Balaji S, Johnson TB, Sade RM, et al: Management of atrial flutter after the Fontan procedure. *J Am Coll Cardiol* 23:1209–1215, 1994.
14. Paul T, Ziemer G, Luhmer I, et al: Atrial arrhythmias after modified Fontan operation: Effect of preoperative hemodynamics and the kind of operation (atriopulmonary vs. total cavopulmonary anastomosis) (in German). *Z Kardiol* 82:368–375, 1993.
15. Cecchin F, Johnsrude CL, Perry JC, et al: Effect of age and surgical technique on symptomatic arrhythmias after the Fontan procedure. *Am J Cardiol* 76:386–391, 1995.
16. Kao JM, Alejos JC, Grant PW, et al: Conversion of atriopulmonary to cavopulmonary anastomosis in management of late arrhythmias and atrial thrombosis. *Ann Thorac Surg* 58:1510–1514, 1994.
17. Vitullo DA, DeLeon SY, Berry TE, et al: Clinical improvement after revision in Fontan patients. *Ann Thorac Surg* 61:1797–1804, 1996.
18. Kreutzer J, Keane JF, Lock JE, et al: Conversion of modified Fontan procedure to lateral atrial tunnel cavopulmonary anastomosis. *J Thorac Cardiovasc Surg* 111:1169–1176, 1996.
19. McElhinney DB, Reddy VM, Moore P, et al: Revision of previous Fontan connections to extracardiac or intraatrial conduit cavopulmonary anastomosis. *Ann Thorac Surg* 62:1276–1282, discussion 1283.

Index